Show Me Where It Hurts

GRAPHIC MEDICINE

Books in the Graphic Medicine series are inspired by a growing awareness of the value of comics as an important resource for communicating about a range of issues broadly termed "medical." For health care practitioners, patients, families, and caregivers dealing with illness and disability, graphic narrative enlightens complicated or difficult experience. For scholars in literary, cultural, and comics studies, the genre articulates a complex and powerful analysis of illness, medicine, and disability and a rethinking of the boundaries of "health." The series includes original comics from artists and nonartists alike, such as self-reflective "graphic pathographies" or comics used in medical training and education, as well as monographic studies and edited collections from scholars, practitioners, and medical educators.

OTHER TITLES IN THE SERIES:

MK Czerwiec, Ian Williams, Susan Merrill Squier, Michael J. Green, Kimberly R. Myers, and Scott T. Smith, *Graphic Medicine Manifesto*

Ian Williams, *The Bad Doctor: The Troubled Life and Times of Dr. Iwan James*

Peter Dunlap-Shohl, *My Degeneration: A Journey Through Parkinson's*

Aneurin Wright, *Things to Do in a Retirement Home Trailer Park . . . When You're 29 and Unemployed*

Dana Walrath, *Aliceheimers: Alzheimer's Through the Looking Glass*

Lorenzo Servitje and Sherryl Vint, eds., *The Walking Med: Zombies and the Medical Image*

Henny Beaumont, *Hole in the Heart: Bringing Up Beth*

MK Czerwiec, *Taking Turns: Stories from HIV/AIDS Care Unit 371*

Paula Knight, *The Facts of Life*

Gareth Brookes, *A Thousand Coloured Castles*

Jenell Johnson, ed., *Graphic Reproduction: A Comics Anthology*

Olivier Kugler, *Escaping Wars and Waves: Encounters with Syrian Refugees*

Judith Margolis, *Life Support: Invitation to Prayer*

Ian Williams, *The Lady Doctor*

Sarah Lightman, *The Book of Sarah*

Benjamin Dix and Lindsay Pollock, *Vanni: A Family's Struggle Through the Sri Lankan Conflict*

Ephameron, *Us Two Together*

Scott T. Smith and José Alaniz, eds., *Uncanny Bodies: Superhero Comics and Disability*

MK Czerwiec, ed., *Menopause: A Comic Treatment*

Susan Merrill Squier and Irmela Marei Krüger-Fürhoff, eds., *PathoGraphics: Narrative, Aesthetics, Contention, Community*

Swann Meralli and Deloupy, *Algériennes: The Forgotten Women of the Algerian Revolution*

Aurélien Ducoudray and Jeff Pourquié, *The Third Population*

Abby Hershler, Lesley Hughes, Patricia Nguyen, and Shelley Wall, eds., *Looking at Trauma: A Tool Kit for Clinicians*

Kimberly R. Myers, Molly L. Osborne, and Charlotte A. Wu, Illustrations by Zoe Schein, *Clinical Ethics: A Graphic Medicine Casebook*

Meredith Li-Vollmer, *Graphic Public Health: A Comics Anthology and Road Map*

Show Me Where It Hurts

Manifesting Illness and Impairment in Graphic Pathography

Monica Chiu

The Pennsylvania State University Press | University Park, Pennsylvania

Library of Congress Cataloging-in-Publication Data

Names: Chiu, Monica, 1965– author.
Title: Show me where it hurts : manifesting illness and impairment in graphic pathography / Monica Chiu.
Other titles: Graphic medicine.
Description: University Park, Pennsylvania : The Pennsylvania State University Press, [2024] | Series: Graphic medicine | Includes bibliographical references and index.
Summary: "Explores graphic pathography, long-form comics by and about subjects who suffer from disease or are impaired, and how it improves various negatively affected corporeal states through hand-drawn images"—Provided by publisher.
Identifiers: LCCN 2023041346 | ISBN 9780271096827 (hardback)
Subjects: LCSH: Graphic medicine (Comic books)—History and criticism. | LCGFT: Comics criticism.
Classification: LCC NC1763.M4 C49 2024 | DDC 741.5/3561—dc23/eng/20230922
LC record available at https://lccn.loc.gov/2023041346

Printed in the United States of America
Published by The Pennsylvania State University Press, University Park, PA 16802–1003

The Pennsylvania State University Press is a member of the Association of University Presses.
It is the policy of The Pennsylvania State University Press to use acid-free paper. Publications on uncoated stock satisfy the minimum requirements of American National Standard for Information Sciences—Permanence of Paper for Printed Library Material, ANSI Z39.48–1992.

For Brian, in sickness and in health

Contents

Illustrations

Acknowledgments

I gratefully acknowledge my many readers, and I apologize to those I might've accidentally overlooked: Jeanette Roan, Stephen Roxburgh, Robin Hackett, Lisa Botshon, Lisa Walker, Siobhan Senier, Melinda Plastas, Rebecca Herzig, Eve Raimon, Carol Conaway, Jana French. I thank an anonymous reader invited by Penn State University Press to comment on the manuscript and Nancy Pedri, the second reader who provided her name for reference, for all of their astute comments that have improved the book. A University of New Hampshire (UNH) Provost's Faculty Fellowship allowed me to work on the manuscript full-time in spring 2022. Funding from UNH's Department of English Gift Account, generously distributed by Professor and Department Chair James Krasner, covered the costs of indexing. To those comics artists and presses that permitted gratuitous use of images from some of the graphic narratives discussed—my gratitude! Acknowledgments are given in the image captions.

Introduction

Making Illness and Impairment Manifest

In health, our sense of inhabiting a body diminishes. We hardly acknowledge our corporality when we are strong, pain free, and psychologically robust. In illness, however, our "ordinary life-in-the-world suddenly collapse[s]," argues Anne Hunsaker Hawkins in her study of prose pathography (2). Atypical sensations caused by disease, impairment, and disability—and sometimes biomedical treatments themselves—remind us of what Drew Leder calls a "recessed body" (36). According to Leder, our inner workings (a pumping heart, a filtering kidney, a digesting stomach) are erased from consciousness until they become dysfunctional. If good health contributes to bodily unconsciousness—somatically "dys-appeared" in unobstructed operation (91)—then illness and biomedicine keenly remind us of our corporeal state. Graphic pathography, or long-form comics by and about subjects who suffer from disease or are impaired,[1] revitalize and re-vision the recessed body in its "dysfunction" through hand-drawn images (69). The formal qualities of comics invite artists to inhabit their bodies as both intimately familiar and as embodied alienation. The artists of graphic pathography necessarily depend on the body to reimagine it on the page. Likewise, the subjects of graphic pathography refuse to concede to the management of their corporeality under clinical, visual organization. By the body and for the body, the medium is subversive and reparative, animating vital images of the self against clinical medicine's static visual archive.[2]

First, this book explores how graphic pathography rematerializes the disappearing body on the comics page.[3] In the institutional maw of clinical medicine that all too often systematizes subjects rather than individualizing them, comics invite innovative techniques of self-representation. Graphic pathography, which falls under the umbrella of graphic medicine (comics broadly about the field of health care), repudiates the biopower of clinical medicine, where positivist knowledge reigns over ambiguity, the latter often overwhelming patients' own encounters with illness and diagnosis. My interpretations explore how artists bestow agency on their cartoon selves through thoughtful depictions of their corporeality drawn against disciplining representations created for them under health care and within health care spaces. We might usefully remind ourselves that the Latin-derived term "patient" is defined as the "quality of being willing to bear adversities; a calm endurance of misfortune; bearing of suffering."[4] Where do we see the un-patient (the not patient subject) of graphic pathography, those characters who unwillingly bear adversity? In the rapidly growing field of autographics[5]—autobiographical comics, including much graphic pathography—if all subjects need their own images, the book asks, what kinds of images, in what drawing styles, does graphic pathography show us?

Second, the project advocates that artists who self-depict, who manifest themselves and their conditions on the page as they perceive them, redeem their disappearing bodies. Medicine as a science, an art, a series of narratives about cure, and an arena of technological advances, is dependent on its collection of dominant images, culturally created, publicly circulated by media, and internalized by patients. Medicine iteratively produces the subjects to which it attends, simplifying care through normative approaches on the one hand, complicating ministration for those who fall beyond its normative purview on the other. Primary sources in the book's chapters visually externalize subjects' conventionally hidden vulnerabilities because they are expected; for example, the sting of stigma surrounding impairment might be agonizingly drawn out, relocating impairment from individual bodies to the cultural realm that shames and stigmatizes those with disabilities. Through comics artists' self-representations, traces of these imputations and even medicine's organizing gaze encounter a slow chipping away, sometimes a complete demolition. Graphic pathography's illustrations revise and revitalize the range of bodily expressions available in the social-medical tableau. As part of broader considerations in the health humanities, this study examines the creative mechanisms by which the subject, renamed as a patient in objective, medical case studies, gains agency in the illustrative practice of self-care. Drawing aslant, or against dominant images of disability and sickness that displace them, the affected person resituates herself into the heart of care.[6] Subjects that look at themselves with compassion look out for themselves. Reclaiming a body interpolated within established images mitigates total dependence on clinical authority's image making.

A third goal is to demonstrate graphic pathography's significant role as a bridge between clinical and autographic envisioning, serving as a literal and metaphorical *medium*. If courses in literature and medicine depend on art, film, poetry, novels, and essays by which to offer alternative, nonbiomedical viewpoints to medical students and health care professionals, my readings invite possibilities for dialogue about graphic pathography created by both patient *and* practicing providers. Each party arrives at the clinical encounter with various narratives and expectations. How can their similarity of concerns and convergences be addressed? Can "regimes of vision," in Jay Dolmage's words, become visionary regimes, the term "visionary" here expressing that which stands outside the banal, the given, that which prophesizes or indicates other ways of seeing ("Disabled upon Arrival" in *Cultural Critique* 27)? The conclusion advocates for medical interns' self-care, through autographic comics about their experiences, as they circulate in the same hierarchical, clinical environment encompassing their patients. I ask, if graphic medicine advances lessons for clinicians, what do comics by and about medical students and practicing clinicians, like MK Czerweic, who is known as the comics nurse, provide for the layperson? Anne Whitehead and Angela Woods pose foundational questions: "How might the bodies of doctors and patients be marked in terms of race, class, gender, ability and disability, and to what effects? What else, we might ask, is in the room? [Or how, I ask in chapter 4, is the clinical space of hospital waiting rooms configured and to what outcome?] . . . And with what forms or modes of agency might marked bodies be associated? How might we account for non-human objects and presences?" (2; a discussion of the latter, on vibrant materialism, is the content of chapter 6). We find "equivocal meanings" in comics, contends Ian Williams ("Comics and the Iconography of Illness" 132). How might these ambiguities resonate among patients as they move from health care practitioners' education—academic lessons in compassion and cultural competence—into their daily practice?

Throughout the study, I highlight challenges to equity proposed by graphic pathography's often quite subtle advancement of social justice solutions to health care challenges. The book follows on the heels of Susan Merrill Squier and Irmela Marei Krüger-Fürhoff's edited collection *PathoGraphics*, a broad examination of how graphic pathography communicates life writing and extends the field of graphic medicine to include social justice health issues related to environmentalism and anthropomorphic effect bound up with molecular affect.[7] Wedded to the ethics of what is right and compassionate for everybody, social justice inquiries include the following: Who has been permitted excellent treatment and who has been left to languish? Who falls ill more frequently and why?[8] Which bodies are regarded as "naturally" insufficient and weak, and how does that designation play out in society, health care? Through revelations of inequalities and subsequent changes to language, laws, and public policy, social justice perspectives advocate universal corrections to conditions that pathologize, that limit, and that far too frequently overlook particular (raced) bodies. That the collected phalanx of comics provides reparative depictions gestures usefully and necessarily to wider challenges in need of social, legal, and political solutions.

Taken up explicitly in chapter 6, "Vital Viruses: Animating Herpes, Pathologizing Whiteness in Dahl's *Monsters* and Schulz's *Sick*," and extended in the coda, I repudiate the absence of graphic pathography by and about people of color. Whose dysfunctional body is most often featured in the medium? If predominantly white bodies self-represent, what does this glaring omission portend for the larger field of graphic medicine and its readers? To whom does medicine cater? Historically, black men and women unknowingly served as experimental bodies for medical science; meanwhile, Asian immigrant bodies were grounded in cultural narratives of both disease and palliation, the former playing out currently during the COVID virus pandemic, the latter in their consideration as model minorities. In what unfortunate ways do images of black, yellow, and brown bodies intersect with illness and disability? How is an academic focus on comics by white subjects consciously exposing or unconsciously contributing to a historical convergence among race, disease, and disability?

Show Me Where It Hurts is the second monograph dedicated explicitly to graphic pathography. Elisabeth El Refaie's *Visual Metaphor and Embodiment in Graphic Illness Narratives* is the first, in which she references over thirty graphic illness narratives "to develop the concept of dynamic embodiment" and "search for patterns of metaphor" (12). While I centralize theme-based, close readings of specific graphic narratives, she focuses on how conceptual metaphor theory (CMT) assists in conveying abstract states of being, "such as mental states, emotions, and social relations, that are hard for us to grasp and convey to others without recourse to our 'embodiment'" (1). El Refaie may have chosen from many genres in the medium to exemplify how CMT works. My study, however, depends on graphic pathography to argue its case; it is geared toward unique interpretations based on specific graphic pathographies. However, I reference El Refaie's work throughout.

Graphic pathography is a new but growing field within the umbrella of graphic medicine, the latter an apt neologism coined by a fierce advocate of the medium of graphic pathography, Ian Williams. Suffering from mental health issues himself, he explains graphic medicine as illustrating subjects in the process of "owning our own conditions" and "reclaim[ing]" our body "from the hands of the healthcare professionals" ("Comics and the Iconography of Illness" 132). Through unexpected methodologies of affect theory, spatial theory, vital materialism, and using approaches from race and ethnic studies, women and gender studies, disability studies, and comics studies, I provide readings of recently published graphic pathography, as well as those that receive little scholarly attention; I offer fresh interpretations of some oft-discussed texts. Rather than filling the proverbial scholarly gap, I interrogate obligatory self-care through graphic pathography's self-manifestations, discuss the relevance of racial absences, exercise the uses of materialism, delve into the possibilities of reparative comics collaborations, and examine built and constructed space as critical medical-cultural territory.

Making Illness Manifest

In Kathryn Montgomery Hunter's *Doctors' Stories: The Narrative Structure of Medical Knowledge*, the patient's story of illness that is presented to the physician is retold through clinical diagnosis. It returns to the patient, from the doctor, in a language she cannot fathom, distancing her from her own body and from a valuable professionally intimate relationship with her physician.[9] In graphic pathography, patients turn clinical narratives into images of the *soma* that imagine against this returned, often incomprehensible, medical perspective. Graphic pathography specifically draws out what an affected or afflicted subject sees and feels that is untethered from or in contrast to medical diagnosis and clinical-visual knowledge. *Drawing*, as both noun and verb, is an essential component of this study whose primary sources rely on the somatic: graphic pathography's hand is the illustrating agent of the sick body. At the same time, a body in sickness might be kinesthetically obstructed from crafting its own representation, from drawing out what illness looks like.

"Hand" is not only an appendage that creates a work of art but also a comics moniker for artistic style. With and through the hand, graphic pathographies make illness manifest. That which manifests, or which aesthetically captures depictions of the afflicted and the attention of its reader, is made apparent on the page. "Manifest," defined as obvious, disclosed, evident, and shown, is derived from the Latin terms "*manus*" for hand and "*(in)festus*," to attack or to irritate, as in an infestation (or infection) that troubles the body. Literally, "manifest" is to be struck with the hand. Williams usefully divides graphic pathography's "ways of showing" into three categories. "The Concealed" are conditions like herpes, where the virus may lie dormant for years or may not present in visible places on the body ("Comics and the Iconography of Illness" 119). "The Invisible" includes mental illnesses, which are not evident on the skin but "are felt or produce psychological suffering" (119). And "The Manifest," which is defined as "the signs of illness or the scars of treatment [that] are visibly scripted on the body" (119). Illnesses trouble the body, while their subsequent creative depiction on the page move their readers—they are struck by the artist's hand.

Finally, because graphic pathographies are hand-drawn representations recording illness or impairment, they are akin to ships' manifests, logs or journals documenting passengers and cargo, while manifestations can refer to emotions or spiritual feelings rendered visible or public. For this reason, authors of *Graphic Medicine Manifesto* locate their work at the "intersection of the medium of comics and the discourse of healthcare" (Czerwiec, Williams et al. 10). This study is about the hand-making manifestation of—the rendering discernable, perceivable, apparent, and visible—the reappearing (once dys-appeared) body in illness, disease, pain, impairment, and disability, all terms fully defined below.

Artistic depictions of illness are not new. In the modernist era, Pablo Picasso's Blue Period conveyed notions of melancholy while *avant garde* work depicting mental illness, such as productions by Leonardo da Vinci and Leon Battista Alberti, conveyed profoundly personal images in a recognizable style. For David Rosand, an artist's line is "both work and signature" (7), a type of protagonist "establishing its own reciprocal relationship with its maker" (12).[10] Comics art, however, is distinguished from painting, and from the culture of film for that matter, through word-image sequentialism, whose properties capitalize on movement and stasis, various self-representations depicted separately and at once, among other affordances used throughout this study.[11]

In graphic pathography, the illustrating hand is an embodied, interpretive tool crafting somatic representations of the state of being unwell, incapacitated, or otherwise enabled. For example, "The hand is a long-established point of intersection between art and medicine," states Ludmilla Jordanova ("Medicine and the Visual Arts" 47). Additionally, in one of Hillary Chute's earliest essays on graphic narrative, she defines the medium as a "subjective register" of comics' materialism in which "the presence of the body, through the hand, [i]s a mark in the text" ("Comics as Literature?" 457). She argues in a subsequent publication that "marks on the page "are an "index of the body"

("Comics Form and Narrating Lives" 112).[12] In *Graphic Embodiments*, editors Lisa DeTora and Jodi Cressman argue that graphic narrative is an "embodied . . . practice" that inform us "about embodied conditions of well-being" (16, 15). And El Refaie claims that "the traces left by the hand of the artist that moves over the page at a particular tempo and rhythm" are, quoting Tim Ingold, "both inspired by, and carry forth, our affective lives" (El Refaie 140). As these scholars claim, graphic pathography illustrates the inseparability between the body and what ails it, drawing out not only a patient's public face but also what illness looks like—the face it publicly presents. The hand as style captures our attention. It can also strike us when it troubles accepted notions of how illness is embodied. Articulate images invite us to see through the lens of illness: What does it mean to be infirm in relation to ourselves, whether healthy or sick, and under the auspices of society's own determinations of what it means to be healthy, to be well? They encourage related queries into illness and perception, such as how do we valuably recognize and compassionately care for the ailing?[13]

Nate Powell's *Swallow Me Whole* provides an initial example of such an intervention. The graphic pathography depicts the ghosts, insects, and wizards that are the hallucinatory manifestations of two stepsiblings' childhood schizophrenia. In sharp black pen strokes on white paper, Powell materializes for his readers the psychological conjuring of apparitions perceptible only to the teen protagonists, Perry and Ruth. Powell's drawn versions of the youths' visions make discernible the indiscernible, enabling our own vision from a literal, perceptible *view*-point. The teens are not "crazy" but untreated; they are not obstreperous but rather ignorant of what afflicts them. Powell's graphic narrative is informed by a decade of his own work among adults with developmental disabilities.[14] *Swallow Me Whole* demonstrates how those who live and circulate among the ill, as well as patients who live in the kingdom of the sick (in reference to Susan Sontag), might valuably *image* their conditions of literal and psychological pain against medical prescriptions circumscribing their health. The psychologist in *Swallow Me Whole*, for example, does not explain Ruth's "obsessive compulsive disorder" or "schizophrenic and dissociative patterns," neither to Ruth nor to her mother, instead handing over an illegible prescription (n.p.). After Perry confesses to his physician that "I hear this little guy [a wizard in Powell's drawings] who follows me around and makes me draw," the latter dismissively tells his father, "The kid is clearly a wizard. He just needs to have the time to focus on his work there. Off you go. A few problems are always normal. Where would we be without them?" (n.p.). Ruth unexpectedly takes flight in one of her hallucinations. In a strange and unexpected drawing, she drifts freely down the street in stark contrast to the insects—that are meant to fly—that she has trapped in labeled jars and collected in her bedroom. We conjecture that she has been overcome by mental illness. I contend, therefore, that drawing in graphic pathography is clearly a disruption, a slap of the hand, a handy slap, a (drawing) hand that presents invisible manifestations of illness to render them image-able and imaginable. Graphic pathography like Powell's can show us where it hurts.

Definitions and Demarcations: Impairment, Agency, Social Justice

I use three terms that require definitions in the context of my work: disability (including its interactions with impairment and its necessary distancing from illness and disease), agency, and social justice. I adhere to a social theory model of disability, briefly outlined here, but also am persuaded by Elizabeth Barnes's "mere-difference" view of disability, what she deems a minority among a minority, explained below.[15] Megan Strickfaden's inquiry—at what point does visual impairment cross the "threshold" into disability?—introduces the gray area surrounding what the nondisabled mean by the term disability (161).[16] Eyeglasses remedy "acceptable vision loss," she argues. "Acceptable," I assume, because so many depend on corrective lenses (161). Thus, in the ubiquity of "acceptable vision loss," eyeglasses both can correct commonly experienced impairment and serve as fashion statements. That is, while restoring acceptable vision loss, we also can choose from an astounding array of stylish frames. Or, we can merely enhance our wardrobe with fake (noncorrective) lenses inserted into trendy frames—wherein some might choose disability's "correction" absent of the impairment. If many people are limited by nearsightedness or farsightedness, or experience "acceptable vision loss," remediation is rendered attractive, even desirable. Fashion surrounding this type of acceptable impairment forces us to ask who defines "acceptable" and what does that definition portend for those with "unacceptable" impairments—Strickfaden's "extreme vision loss" (161)—those we might not select for ourselves? What does this distinction mean in disability studies and for disability activists? The terms on which medicine has settled ("extreme vision loss" chafes against "acceptable vision loss") determine the conditions upon which the abled and those personally limited (in motion, cognitively, in vision) view themselves, rather than allowing the conditions to set the determinants.

Disability studies scholar Christopher Bell reminds us of the ever-changing domain of terms and arguments by which we define "disability," noting how in the past some, but not all, scholars in the field once regarded AIDS as a disability; others find that those "with hidden disabilities" are not sufficiently disabled ("Introduction: Doing Representational Detective Work" 3). Conferring or denying the designation "disabled," as we know, has implications for insurance coverage, for obtaining specific procedures or medications, for receiving unemployment benefits, for being granted a designated vehicle tag permitting parking in specific spots, and opens disabled subjects to social stigma.

In disability studies, those who embrace a social theory model over a medical one argue that the built environment prevents disabled subjects from mobility, sometimes from social and educational advancement.[17] To call disability a "political category," Susan Wendell argues, places the burden on social, material conditions that impose barriers to those so named: disability in this social theory model is "the socially constructed disadvantage based upon impairment" (22).[18] Similarly, Simi Linton argues that disability is a term derived from and conferring significance to the medical community, in which "human variation" in the form of impairment is regarded "as deviance from the norm, as pathological condition, as deficit" (11). Yet to be limited in mobility or to necessitate assistance to function in an ableist world does not require a cure.[19] Thus ascribing illness to disability, as mutually constitutive, is perniciously "problematic," argues Wendell (17). "To cure something implies that you are returning the body to its normal state," claims Emily Ladau. "[However,] my disability *is* my normal state" (quoted in Elizabeth Barnes 143).

A third view between the medical model and the social model is that of the interactionalist model, laid out by Christopher Riddle. This third outlook neither dismisses the medical model nor totally embraces the social model but insists that approaches mediated by both will best ameliorate pain and any limitations, built and social, impeding the impaired. Constructing a built environment facilitating mobility for an individual with an amputation, for example, might improve her mobility, but this built solution alone does not address residual discomfort. "Impairments must necessarily have negative impacts for individuals," states Riddle, "otherwise, we do not consider the social oppression resulting from the condition as disability at all" (Riddle paraphrases John Harris 35). If illness seeks a cure, so, too, does disability in this coterminous but maligned association as, returning to Landau, "My disability *is* my normal state." As many scholars in a social theory model of disability studies advocate then, "It is ableism [as a deliberately normalizing structure] that needs the cure, not our bodies" (Eli Clare quoted in Wendell 18).

Finally, I turn to Elizabeth Barnes, whose thought-provoking philosophical approach to disability in *The Minority Body: A Theory of Disability*, systematically unpacks and carefully overturns many standard arguments used by disability scholars in order to advance a "mere-difference" view of disability. In this extremely truncated definition, absent of Barnes's valuable nuances, "disability is *neutral* with regard to well-being" (emphasis in original 54).[20] Disability "makes you *different*," she claims, renders a person a minority among other minorities, but does not intrinsically make them "worse off"; the disabled as "worse off" is an assessment held by those adhering to "bad-difference views" of disability (54, 55). She relies on testimony from disabled subjects to make her claims, which I find most helpful when sifting through various definitions of and approaches to disability. For in our ableist world, we have practiced "testimonial injustice," which impedes those of a minority group from being listened to (135), while "hermeneutical injustice" inhibits them from recognizing and expressing their experiences because of reigning stigmas about disability (169).[21] Following Barnes's valuable explorations of both these forms of "epistemic injustice" (169), I contend that the autographic subjects addressed in *Show Me Where It Hurts* resist what I call visual injustice. Sometimes they depict challenges they confront in the built environment, other times are thwarted by social judgment, but finally draw out, with joy, embodied agency.

The impairment/disability divide has a corollary in that of illness/disease. "Impairment" for some scholars is a subject's social experience with (the medical model of) disability. Likewise, illness, according to Arthur Kleinman, is "the innately human experiences of symptoms and suffering" of disease, where disease is the term given to a medical condition whose symptoms, signs, prognoses, and possible cures are mapped scientifically on the body, over time (4). "Disease is what practitioners have been trained to see," he claims (5). Illness is a subject's response to disease, the uncharted territory of how disease "feels" to the ill. Turning again to the often (harmful) intertwining of illness and impairment, we are reminded that some impaired subjects are not well. A woman who has lost a limb from diabetes, for example, is hospitalized for pneumonia, only to be discharged once cleared of the latter. But she will not be admitted for and cured of her amputation, unless it becomes infected.[22] Some illnesses become temporarily disabling. Others, such as those that are chronic, can be permanently disabling. I will use illness and impairment as subjects' embodied experiences, disease and disability as their denoted medical conditions.

In my analysis, subjects of graphic pathography defined by the medical model of disease and disability both desire and then draw their agency beyond the bounds of the constructed, normative patient. I turn to Judith Butler's definition of agency as constrained by sex and gender yet still open to liberation as explored in *Bodies That Matter*. She revisits and more expansively defines agency, taken up as performativity in her poststructural study *Gender Trouble*. Critiques of agency in performativity contend that in Butler's definition of gender, subjects that are bound to obligatory codes can react only within the codes' confines. The conditions that create the subject are the same conditions that bind her. Therefore, there exists no woman before or beyond that construction, argues Adriana Zaharijević (25). Clinical medicine's discursive management of the body around narrow definitions of well-being limns the enigma that Butler's critics allege: Is Butler's performative subject agential? Is any cure for an already prescribed subject anything but a prescriptive one?[23]

In *Bodies That Matter*, Butler replies to her critics by explaining that the regulatory codes constraining sex and gender also are the very social codes that will afford opportunities beyond codification. Bodies produced under "regulatory schemas" also produce the possibilities of that which is unregulated, that which might be "unimaginable" (Butler xi). The construction of sex or gender does not foreclose its complete submission to a regulating power. The performativity of gender, she argues, as repetitive processes of acting within discursive or social norms, might also be "sites of critical agency" (x).[24] I extend Butler's understanding of agency in discussing how subjects of graphic pathography are hindered by medical dispositions, exemplified by rigid narratives of cure and under a limited set of images (or rephrased as a limited imagination). Under what circumstances might a patient invoke her own agency? She may initially internalize the medical approach, I argue, but in becoming a self-conscious agent able and willing to act on intentions, she re-signifies medical codes in her drawings.[25]

While it is beyond the scope of this book to explore the historical and political genealogy of social justice, as well as new liberalism's notions of social justice,[26] brief definitional guidelines are appropriate. Walter Lorenz helpfully explains that the term social justice "has come to refer commonly to social policies and other rights-based initiatives that protect vulnerable and disadvantaged groups of national or global society from oppression, discrimination, or exclusion or that support them materially" (14). He distinguishes between an "entitlement" aspect of social justice and "charitable approaches" (15). The former advances that no matter one's identity (race, gender, sexual orientation, economic class, religion, or faith), citizens are authorized, by law, to equitable services. In "charitable approaches," various governing or social bodies decide who deserves what rights, to what extent and quality, and so define who might be deprived of them. Subjects in the primary texts I explore turn to entitlement approaches.

Loretta Capeheart and Dragan Milovanovic also usefully define social justice as a community endeavor, as that beyond "what is just for the individual alone" to "what is just for the social whole" (2). Social justice is a "we" problem. Consider the sixty-four comics published in *COVID Chronicles: A Comics Anthology*, which addresses "how the actions of an invisible microbe," states the collection's editor Kendra Boileau, resulted in "systemic upheaval" (xi). The virus may have overwhelmed our institutions of medicine, collapsed much of the economy, and iterated clearly the chasms of care in the seeming bedrock of American social justice, but it also uncannily has forged connections and community, she continues (xi). As such, throughout this study I inquire: When self-care burgeons into care of all selves, what does graphic pathography's imaging mean beyond the individual? How do resistant, multiple (rather than singular), changing (over static) views inform the institution particularly and social and cultural arenas broadly?

The Medical Humanities' Narrative Medicine, the Health Humanities' Graphic Pathography

In their introduction to *Infertility Comics and Graphic Medicine*, Chinmay Murali and Sathyaraj Venkatesan comprehensively chart the field of comics and graphic medicine, from the medical humanities[27] to its more expansive health humanities.[28] The latter incorporates findings in women and gender studies, queer studies, race and ethnic studies, and disability studies;[29] and by acknowledging the wide swath of caregivers beyond physicians and nurses, such as paid caregivers who attend to patients in their homes; "informal caregivers," including family members; and those who make care possible, such as "charitable organizations' personnel; paraprofessionals and support staff; custodial servicers; and ambulance staff" (Paul Crawford et al. 12). While the medical humanities often have focused on the clinical side of wellness and targeted the contributions of medical staff, the health humanities, which encompass critical medical humanities, engage the social sciences, arts, and humanities, and provide pedagogical tools for all caregivers invested in redefining health for the benefit of the ill.

In Murali and Venkatesan's overview of the rise of graphic medicine, they advocate for a convergence of ideas as they emerged over time as opposed to a linear, chronological trajectory from narrative medicine to the health humanities to graphic medicine.[30] Comics, they argue, have been in existence long before the health humanities itself. In the history to follow—of the interaction among the medical humanities, the health humanities, and graphic medicine—I am indebted to Murali and Venkatesan's very thorough charting of the rise of graphic pathography. I necessarily revisit some of that territory but ultimately expand the base by filling in some gaps and finding new avenues to explore.

Medical education was, since 1948, "multidisciplinary" to its core, Murali and Venkatesan remind us (16), and even by 1937, they refine, E. E. Reinke of the Vanderbilt School of Medicine advocated for a medical/technical education hand in hand "with a liberal education" (17). The value to medical practice of studies in language, culture, and the social sciences eventually led to related courses in medical programs, and those initial offerings, including a history of medicine, began to populate the curriculum of the first medical humanities department, launched in 1967, at Penn State University's Hershey Medical Center.

Literature and medicine, a branch of clinical studies, relies on the arts and humanities to instruct thoughtful attention to patients and the cultivation of empathy. The culture of medicine, not the "hard" experiential positivism of the sciences, aligned closely with the interpretative skills of other disciplines; physicians' thoughtful readings of signs, emotions, and signals given by the patient and her body assumed a valued adjunct to careful somatic reading and cultivated respectful bedside manner. Literature and medicine was established in its academic form in 1972, when Joanne Trautmann (Banks) accepted a position teaching literature at Penn State University College of Medicine (Hawkins and McEntyre 4). The emergence of the interdisciplinary journal *Literature and Medicine*, published by Johns Hopkins University Press, confirmed the field's academic acceptance (4). These literary additions contribute, they imagine (but have yet to be decisively proven, as assessed in the conclusion), to capacious, competent care.

Early iterations of the introduction of narrative medicine to health care are attributed to Rita Charon, who holds both an MD and a PhD in English. She encouraged her colleagues in Columbia University's medical school to introduce students to narrative competence using novels. In 2000, Charon persuasively argued that literature and literary representations of illness, disease, suffering, and recovery are essential reading for those studying the biological human condition.[31] For example, Leo Tolstoy's 1886 *The Death of Ivan Ilych*, in which Ivan, confined to his deathbed, desperately wishes to be acknowledged as a thinking and feeling human being by the doctor who is overseeing his illness while seeing over, ignoring, his patient (*Narrative Medicine* 22–23).[32] Clinical effectiveness, Charon claims, is grounded in reading many types of narratives, not only the trajectory of illness in a body but also patient in-takes, test results, physicians' reports, the somatic body and its many signs (including emotions). Learning to interpret literature is key to Charon's advocacy of practicing good medicine, as we all tell stories about ourselves and our bodies, especially in the clinic (*Narrative Medicine*).

Other academic fields, such as the behavioral sciences, medical sociology, and medical anthropology, gradually enriched a changing medical curriculum. The health humanities, or wider yet still a "health studies" field that incorporates approaches from both the medical humanities and the health humanities, is incontrovertibly interdisciplinary.[33] For those working in the broad health care field, caring for humans and understanding the human condition involves much more than knowledge in the sciences, mathematics, and attending to illness and disease during internships and rotations. "The majority of healthcare as it is practised is non-medical," claim the editors of the 2015 collection *Health Humanities* (Crawford et al. 2).

Those afflicted with illness in a purely clinical setting long for somebody to ask, "What's it like?" or to solicit a patient's perspective, as does Tolstoy's Ivan. In the 1990s, prose illness pathographies began to provide such a perspective in a general deviance from and critique of those narratives produced by clinical medicine. These written accounts allow the "ill to tell their own stories," "a need for a voice they can recognize as their own" (Frank 3, 7). For Einat Avrahami, "Bodies are a source of knowledge" (66), and thus "illness narratives are political agents for change insofar as they allow sick and disabled people to break the sanction of silence and bring their experiences of cultural oppression to the level of discursive consciousness" (42).[34] Avrahami quotes Christina Middlebrook: "Generations speak different languages. So do people with cancer. We use the same words but we must have different dictionaries. Things I say seem unintelligible to people who live outside the cancer realm. . . . You can only speak the language by living there" (Avrahami 65). Hawkins defines pathography as "a form of autobiography or biography that describes personal experiences of illness, treatment, and sometimes death" (*Reconstructing Illness* 1). Pathography provides the patient a voice rarely heard in the "world of medicine," and it does so in such a way as "to assert the phenomenological, the subjective, and the experiential side of illness," she argues (12).

Graphic pathography, long-form comics by and about those who are ill, respond to "What's it like?" with "Let me show you." Approaches in both narrative and graphic narrative demonstrate how patients seeking medical care refuse to submit to established clinical narratives; they refute others' metaphors if "they lack empathy," according to El Refaie (34), and resist others' retelling of their own stories. If ill people "*need* . . . to tell their stories, in order to construct new maps and new perceptions of their relationships to the world," argues Arthur Frank (3), then I argue that ill subjects also desire their own images.[35] Graphic pathography hosts a telling line and constitutes a visual catalyst. As prose literature bridged the physician's approach to a patient's "words, gestures, silences" (Charon quoted in Murali and Venkatesan 20), artists' aesthetic lines manifest their own views of embodied states. They show us where it hurts.

If clinical medicine participates in the *business* of cure, graphic medicine promotes self-care.[36] The former mandates a financial bottom line. The latter retrieves and rehabilitates the individual subject from the "patient," an illustrated rebuke. Likewise, Eszter Szép in *Comics and the Body: Drawing, Reading, and Vulnerability* addresses not only how the mark-making artist uses her hand, an embodied reaction to depicted vulnerability, but also how the reading body performs "kinaesthetic empathy" (a term she borrows from Laura Marks; see Szép 137). Szép argues for the "performative and embodied nature" of reading comics (139), what she calls "feeling the line" (141).[37] While Szép studies the reader's "reception of abstract lines" (137), I focus on what the line depicts about the institutions of health and medicine for the drawing subject. Szép's conclusion, however, that graphic narratives about the body can convey characters' vulnerability resonates with my exploration of graphic pathography's social justice objectives, indicating which subjects are cared for, how and why, and which ones are less well served by systems of "health" and "care."

Cartoons depicting illness precede the rise of narrative medicine and the health humanities. In *Disability in Comic Books and Graphic Narratives*, Zach Whalen, Chris Foss, and Jonathan Gray find that in the nineteenth century, Britain's weekly publication *Punch* used caricatures of the Irish to depict racial and bodily differences that deviated from the British norm ("Introduction" 3). In the coda, I explore the attribution of disease to race in the immigration history of the United States in relation to the lack of a robust collection of graphic pathography by and about people of color. According to Jared Gardner, graphic illness has always resided in early American cartoon panels; the institutionalization of the health humanities has neglected a heretofore alliance between cartoons and illness. In his keynote address "Beyond Metaphor," for the 2015 Graphic Medicine Conference, Gardner usefully explores the many references to illness featured in Richard Outcault's 1865 Sunday supplement *Hogan's Alley*, considered America's first comic. Gardner singles out the shaven head of the character Yellow Kid, who lives in a lively New York City immigrant neighborhood, as a "prophylactic" against the scourge of lice. Gardner surmises that a smooth pate was a cheap and convenient remedy by which to repel the recurrence of the pesky parasite in a packed neighborhood where eggs pass with ease from hairy head to hairy head. In his accompanying PowerPoint presentation, Gardner compares the likeness of the cartoon Kid to an early-twentieth-century photograph of a child with nutrition deficiency, visually demonstrating how the facial features and bald crowns of Outcault's other cartoon kids indicated a possible widespread alimentary paucity.[38] Furthermore, yellow journalism, a type of reportage suggesting sensationalism, originated in the tug-of war between former newspaper moguls William Randolph Hearst and Joseph Pulitzer over the rights to Outcault's work, an ugly public squabble that gave rise to the name yellow journalism. The Yellow Kid is associated not only with illness as argued by Gardner—being jaundiced or exhibiting the pallor of the sick—but also with the hyperbolic.

Gardner's instructive history of the origins of comics as intertwined with pathology concludes where many other comics scholars' similar trajectories begin: with Justin Green's 1972 *Binky Brown and the Holy Virgin Mary*, once considered the first American graphic pathography, which depicts obsessive compulsive disorder.[39] For Murali and Venkatesan, comics like *Binky Brown* "flourished in the 1960s following comics censorship . . . as it foregrounded the messy and obscene aspects of corporeality, paving the way for honest depictions of illness and suffering in comics" (15). Their reference to underground artists Aline Kominsky-Crumb's 1972 "Goldie: A Neurotic Woman," published in the same year as *Binky Brown*, assists us in rethinking the gendering of the comics canon in its hierarchizing of men's works over women's. Repeated academic attention to *Binky Brown* over scant remembrance of "Goldie" runs parallel to hierarchies of the clinical arena, and to so many other social, cultural establishments, whereby the white male body (here in clinical testing) serves as the universal body; its reactions to drug trials are the harbingers of expected, similar reactions in—and often harmfully erroneous reception by—the bodies of white females and people of color. While the Underground comix movement may have been short-lived, state Murali and Venkastesan, it facilitated the ability for women, decades after, to draw their autobiographical experiences of sexism, violation, homophobia, and emotional distress. Autobiographical comics by women, contends Chute, place pressure "on conceptions of the unrepresentable" by rendering that which was once considered taboo visible on the page (*Graphic Women* 2). Trauma and its attendant disruption to mental wellness are such taboo subjects illustrated in graphic pathography.

One need not look far to find numerous examples of graphic pathography long before its current nomenclature. Ian Williams lists the long-running *Rex Morgan, M.D.* series, in print for over half a century since its 1948 inception, as well as comics biographies about medical figures (such as Louis Pasteur or Florence Nightingale), and comics featuring doctors and nurses based on "real-life medical situations" ("Portrayal of Illness" 65, 66). Similarly, Bert Hansen discusses the ubiquity of "medical history stories" in the genre of American true-adventure comics of the 1940s, such as *True Comics, Real Heroes, Real Life Comics* (179, 180). While he focuses on image styles that, he argues, sustain readerly interest, his emphasis on stories about the lives of actual physicians, nurses, and medical scientists falls within the umbrella of graphic medicine. More recently, Emmanuel Guibert (artist), Didier Lefèvre (photographer), and Frédéric Lemercier (colorist) record character Didier's photographic journey with a medical caravan in *The Photographer: Into War-Torn Afghanistan with Doctors Without Borders*. The graphic pathography and war narrative elegantly juxtapose cartoons and photographs, while also contrasting beautiful landscape against horrific war wounds suffered by soldiers and civilians alike. Marek Bennett tackles Civil War history in *The Civil War Diary of Freeman Colby, 1863* (in two volumes), especially that of nurse Sarah Low and incorporates the literary work of Walt Whitman, penned after visiting Civil War patients in Washington DC–based hospitals (Marek Bennett, vol. 2, appendices 499). Based on letters, diaries, maps, photographs, and other archival information that Bennett perused in local historical societies and libraries around his New Hampshire–based hometown, his work demonstrates an innovative comics approach to war history, biography (of nurses, poet-volunteers), and field hospital experiences of patients and caregivers.

In the realm of superheroes, Ramzi Fawaz examines the initial inclusion of disability and its constructive work in the comics *The Justice League of America*. He argues that it is the first instance in which the League acts individually to solve "threats to their bodily integrity" rather than as a collective, as when they destroy "menaces to international security" (62). For Fawaz, disability resides as nearly insurmountable for these heroes, a feat more challenging than fighting aliens. The *Fantastic Four* emerging in the 1960s, however, introduced superheroes endowed with psychological weaknesses, says Robert Harvey, followed by similarly affected superheroes in the X-Men and the Avengers (47). The *Fantastic Four* battled neuroses whose genesis lay in their expectations of "gender and sexual conformity," argues Fawaz (77). Character Benjamin Grimm, who morphs into The Thing, eventually finds pleasure in his "productively maladjusted stance toward contemporary gender and sexual norms" (Fawaz 77). Emotions such as feeling uncertain or unsettled become positive attributes in the comics universe, especially for superheroes (16). That is, claims Fawaz, the transformed team wrestled an *accidental* biopower charge of a cosmic ray into positive features, hence reworking generations of provocatively termed "mad" scientists in the comics world who *intentionally* injected themselves with power serums.

Senescence also unexpectedly intrudes into the "super" realm of superheroes. This natural, human trajectory encouraged anxiety, and produced accompanying frailty, in characters unnaturally (and assumed perpetually) strong. The retired but eventually revitalized Batman of Frank Miller's *Batman: The Dark Night Returns*, repudiates the reality of growing old. He reluctantly acknowledges the aches and pains of his increasingly stiff and sluggish body, pummeled by years as a superhero who fights with his fists. His face is lined, his confidence shaky, so unlike his younger, irrepressible, and elastic self. When necessary, however, he finds his senior sea legs in order to roundly whip Superman, now a silver-haired superhero himself. Miller's depictions of a resuscitated Batman supports a common human fantasy that bodies, by sheer will, can spurn corporeal and cognitive changes, and often impairments, of "silver," both as seniority and as nomenclature, where the Silver Era itself marks one of various chronological generations in the superhero universe.[40] Alternately, the cover of José Alaniz's scholarly work *Death, Disability, and the Superhero: The Silver Age and Beyond* features a still from Gilles Barbier's 2002 museum installation *Nursing Home*, in which Superman supports himself with a walker, Captain America lies prone on a gurney, while Wonder Woman tends to his intravenous drip (3). These mellowing superheroes are too fragile and sick to face the next major attack on America. Alaniz argues that as images of imperfect bodies pervaded post–World War II American consciousness, known and new superheroes became less and less physically resilient.

My book does not analyze superhero comics, nor does it investigate medical pedagogical comics, the latter an additional genre that falls under graphic pathography. Ian Williams, though, investigates how the influence of AIDS on society in the 1980s and 1990s ushered in commercial-educational comics about prevention and HIV symptoms that destigmatized the disease and whose profits benefited AIDS charities ("Portrayal of Illness" 72).[41] Williams argues that the artists of these comics depicted "their own concepts of the diseased body" and thus appropriated the negative influence of "'official' iconography that informs society's notion of an illness" (74). "Ecopathographies," so named by Hawkins, also are beginning to circulate within graphic pathography, "warning the rest of us," writes Squier, "that their [the comics artists'] illnesses are the signs and symptoms of much larger problems confronting culture as a whole" (Squier references Hawkins 206). Environmental toxins and climate change as social justice issues, global pathogens and parasites as "agential beings" (Squier 209), and "porous pathographies" that invite comprehension and "ramifications at multiple scales simultaneously" (209, 206) point us in new directions in graphic pathography.

This foray into comics publications that preceded the official nomenclature of "graphic narrative" demonstrates how the many incarnations of comics and medicine encompass a much more complex history than that provided to date and invites further study. As the field of graphic medicine grows, so does it expand how we might reimagine what we mean by "medicine" in the term graphic medicine. Perhaps the specific term "graphic pathography" is an overall misnomer that returns us to a medium examining the life of the pathogen or the disease rather than its more humane focus on the life of patients *with* illness or impairment and the providers who circle around them.[42] In *Show Me Where It Hurts*, I accept Williams's challenge to provide "further scholarly attention" to "the quality and quantity of recent depictions of disease in graphic narrative" ("Portrayal of Illness" 75).[43]

Chapter Outlines

I retreat from former comics scholars' heavy reliance on trauma theory, life writing, and Scott McCloud's *Understanding Comics*, even though the latter provides a useful introduction to the medium through the medium. Additionally, the wide range of subject matter in the selected primary sources—on disability, cancer, aging, the encroachment of disease-related blindness, sexually transmitted diseases, and psychosomatic presentations—prevents the manuscript from falling into the narrow parameters of a study focused only on cancer comics, for example, or closely on anorexia and bulimia, infertility issues, Alzheimer's, among other specific diseases. These are certainly viable approaches, but I find vitality in the great variety of graphic pathography that capaciously draws out the dys-appearing body. In a study that critiques the lack of graphic pathography by and about people of color, I intentionally sought out as much scholarship as possible by scholars of color. Throughout, I also rely heavily on literary, cultural, and comics studies, as opposed to work from education, linguistics, and metaphor, as practiced by other comics scholars.[44] Chapters are arranged to build across interwoven themes and, ironically, to move toward discussing the field's significant lacuna: representations of race by artists of color.

In chapter 1, I address how Al Davison's *The Spiral Cage*, an autographic about white, cisgender, impaired Al, asks us to re-vision the normate.[45] If "medicine is fundamentally narrative . . . and its daily practice is filled with stories," as claims Hunter (5), I investigate how Davison's graphic pathography encourages us to become better readers of comics about impairment, a pedagogical approach to relearning how to read, revising our literacy "normate." His somatic texts are what I call graphic genesis, a concept that contributes to improved literacy about ableism. The various generative versions of *The Spiral Cage*, its successive published incarnations from floppy comics to sturdier editions, comment on comics, bodies, and materiality.

Chapter 2 sets Marisa Acocella Marchetto's *Cancer Vixen* against her subsequent graphic narrative *Ann Tenna*, two works collaboratively interrogating and reinstructing us about how "good" and "bad" (white, cisgender) women patients behave. The latter has found little traction in academia even though, I argue, the two are symbiotically related through illness and vanity. The chapter develops from medical and social scripts circumscribing "disease" and "woman" to charting their affects among outrageous and bold women characters.

Care work of the elderly is the focus of chapter 3, the "good" expected work of (white) women and their (white) daughters, examined through style and haptic drawing in Roz Chaz's *Can't We Talk About Something More Pleasant?* and Joyce Farmer's *Special Exits: A Graphic Memoir*. Perusing the various types of succor provided by daughters to their mothers, and what this care work expects of them, I ask why predominantly women are "forced to care," the title of Evelyn Nakano Glenn's study of global women in the caring workforce, and its consequences. The lack of affordable caregivers and facilities for the elderly—a paucity of spaces of good care—brings us to chapter 4. I explore hospital and clinic waiting rooms through spatial theory, carefully unpacking hospital space in Chris Ware's *Jimmy Corrigan: The Smartest Kid on Earth*, and Phoebe Potts's *Good Eggs*. A hospital's literal spaces in which patients circulate are networks of interrelated emotions as well as part and parcel of the medical industrial complex.

This complex, however, administers to race unevenly. Chapter 5 analyzes Vivian Chong and Georgia Webber's *Dancing After TEN*, in which visible impairment and scars from disease contend with the invisibility of race. Chong's Asian Canadian identity and her impending blindness are put in conversation with the myth of the model minority through James Kyung-Jin Lee's notion of "woundedness." Additionally, because each artist-contributor suffers from vastly different debilitations, one permanent (Chong's blindness) and one temporary (Webber's voicelessness), their artistic collaboration evolves into an exciting suturing of experiences that I call graphting.

The penultimate chapter 6 reads Ken Dahl's *Monsters* about herpes, a condition demanding discussion, thereby deshaming the disease. But herpes also provokes excessive worry for protagonist Ken, a white heterosexual, cisgender man living with a manageable disease. These anxieties over an amendable condition are untenable in relation to Vivian's permanent blindness in *Dancing After TEN*. I read herpes through vital materialism, extending agential qualities to the virus. I take up Squier's request that we "challenge the unconscious assumption that pathography belongs only at the scale of the human being," referencing necessarily articulate "spaces between human lives, showing the intimate entanglements that link all human beings not just to each other but also to the other 99 percent of biodiversity and to the earth" ("Scaling Graphic Medicine" 221). I eventually link the monsters of the herpes simplex virus to more unwieldy, less remedied beasts embedded in the privileges and their consequences afforded by racial whiteness. As a logical corollary, *Sick*, a subsequent graphic narrative by Dahl (who also goes by Gabby Schulz), charts the path from comics avatar Gabby's (white) ignorance—"wellness" a manifestation of the bliss of oblivion—to his pathological consciousness of white privilege. In this chapter's conclusion, I contrast Ken/Gabby's experiences falling temporarily ill with those of Japanese-Canadian lesbian Kimiko, in remission from breast cancer (from *Kimiko Does Cancer: A Graphic Memoir* by Kimiko Tobimatsu [author] and Keet Geniza [artist]). Gabby recovers, albeit with the burden of whiteness dogging him, but Kimiko, like Vivian in *Dancing After TEN*, can never overcome the stigma of race negatively affecting her ability to secure resources for her treatment and recovery, and nefarious attitudes about race and disease, the coda's topic.

The conclusion points to graphic pathography's solid future in the health humanities. I argue that this genre of comics is a *medium* in two senses of the term: a noun naming its word-image form and an act of bridging, here from physician to patient. I ask how graphic narratives by and about health care workers might inform patients, among other readers, of the challenges, fears, and joys they confront in the hierarchy of medical education and culture. The endeavor assumes comics as a mediator, linking the concerns of health care providers with those of patients in a social justice arena of graphic medicine's "we."

The coda resists the winding down of a conclusion by inviting more comics artists of color to produce images of illness in our nation's historically deterministic relationship between disability and race, disease and race. The sheer number of graphic pathographies by white artists, ranging across mental health, Parkinson's, cancer, Asperger's, epilepsy, anorexia and bulimia, and a myriad of other diseases and disabilities provides a massive archive from which to fashion extended arguments. The paucity of graphic pathography by and about people of color, however, does not offer such a deep and wide swath.[46] I ask, in what ways has medicine, and how have scholars in the medical humanities and disability studies, contributed to this visual injustice, and often visual violence? How might scholars in the medical humanities and disability studies address the challenge? Does the absence of graphic pathography by people of color continue to suggest that medical care is care for white people? If research already demonstrates that the impact of climate change, COVID-19 and its variants, and medical research all more negatively impact the health and well-being of people of color than they do white people, what are the social justice implications of an unwillingness to draw them out? Without them, we will be mired in Dahl's world of *Sick*, a white world in which injustice is itself invalidating. *Show Me Where It Hurts* reads what already has been manifested on the comics page and invites more of what demands expression.

Chapter 1

Graphic Genesis and the Somatic Text

Davison's *The Spiral Cage*

In *The Minority Body: A Theory of Disability*, Elizabeth Barnes states, "The intuitions of the (privileged) majority don't have a particularly good track record as reliable guides to show how we should think about the minority [here an impaired subject], especially when the minority is a victim of stigma and prejudice" (156). Grounded in this claim, I explore manifestations of comics protagonist Al, a white man, in Al Davison's *The Spiral Cage*. Not only does his self-presentation show readers a life of spina bifida and wellness through comics, but it also teaches the unimpaired, or the majority, how to read them. His illustrations pedagogically and rightfully ask the majority to grapple with deciphering meanings as do the minority struggle in an ableist world. He draws against a consistent practice that Barnes calls "testimonial injustice"—a legacy defined by Miranda Fricker—of judging first-person accounts by the impaired as "unreliable" (136). His depiction is instruction. In correctly assuming that majoritarian readers' experiences have fostered unreliable approaches to his embodied self, Davison instructs them otherwise. *The Spiral Cage* dispenses with flat images and prescribed meanings of those living with spina bifida, and of the condition imagined by the majority largely, by proposing impairment as "an engine of innovation and rhetorical invention" (Dolmage and Jacobs 15). Davison's invention is his comics.

They require lessons in reading his innovative visual rhetoric by which to interpret his embodiment.

Davison was born in 1960 in Newcastle, England, with an incomplete formation of the spinal cord. His doctors assumed he would not survive. When he did, they were convinced he would never walk. But he defied medical diagnosis once again by becoming ambulatory. If infants with spina bifida live, which is often not the case, they can experience paralysis of the lower body, as occurred to Al, and complications to the colon and urinary tract. Davison's intellectually and physically rewarding life refutes the general prognosis of spina bifida as fatal and antithetical to living a full life, so calculated by the majority. In *The Spiral Cage*, drawn iterations of Al successfully living with spina bifida are what I call graphic genesis, pedagogical lessons unfolding across each unique comics page informing us, progressively, how to read Davison's graphic narrative against expected approaches to comics literacy. The aesthetic stratagem itself mimics how character Al accesses mobility and self-confidence otherwise in an able-bodied world.

Davison's seemingly disordered arrangement of panels and pages requires us to read *against* Western, prescribed reading modes: our eyes move horizontally and vertically, across and up, backward and forward on the page. This constant disruption to familiar, established literacy reflects Al's exceptional (both anomalous and explicitly atypical) somatic self. Our gradual reading proficiency rehearses his own progressive self-embodiment. In addition, toggling back and forth among his comics representations as infant, toddler, youth, and adult, Davison disrupts an autobiographical trajectory chronologically mapping childhood to adulthood.[1] If comics have a rhythm in which systemic gridding (waffle gridding, for example) bestows the work an even-handed tempo that might be interrupted, for example, by a "loud" and jarring full-page bleed, Davison's consistent syncopation is recognized *as* its regularity, an off-beat cadence emerging as an accepted norm. Davison's visuals thus accomplish the insurmountable, activating the passivity of the material page in concert with animating a minority body once deemed stationary. Davison does not embody a clinically anticipated stagnation (or paralysis) of those born with spina bifida but defies it literally, by which readers access such defiant somaticism aesthetically. Seemingly chaotic, persistent movement is Davison's careful management of his comics project while so many other aspects of his life lie beyond his control. Through imaginative page and panel layouts requiring more than a passing glance to ascertain meaning, he schools us in reading his graphic embodiment.

In this chapter, my arguments build on connections forged between corporeality and graphics (illustrations), relying on disability studies, specifically those contending that the built environment is an impediment to the impaired, and capitalizing on the normative gaze refracted by Al. In the final section, I consider the materiality of the text by arguing that two sturdy hardcover reprints of *The Spiral Cage*, which emerged from an initial floppy comics format that literally disintegrated on the shelves, are material adjuncts to Al's growing physical stability. Through material text and artistic context, what I call Davison's graphic genesis provides fresh approaches to graphic life writing about impairment. Panels asking us to track this way and that, not necessarily forward or upward—directional terms in Western reading practices suggesting progressive (positive) advancement—revises our understanding of disability as regressive in Davison's able hand/style. His graphic pathography generates—engenders, progresses—an approach to impairment for the able-bodied reader.

Adapting to Graphic Genesis

In their introduction to a 2017 special issue of the *Journal of Graphic Novels and Comics*, editors Aidan Diamond and Lauranne Poharec pose key inquiries of "freaked and Othered bodies in comics": "Which bodies are permitted depiction as heroic or innocent . . . and how does their representational embodiment determine their casting?" (407). Davison's corporeal defiance of such casting—refuting standard negative medical prognosis for infants with spina bifida, including a very early death—mirror Davison's graphic vacillations, visual disruptions to governed reading and looking practices.[2] This includes impeding the narrative trajectory of "traditional male autobiographies [that] search for a true self, present a chronological, linear and ejaculatory narrative structure" (McIlvenny referencing David Jackson 240). Davison does not relate a before- and after-illness story, the "otherwise" narrative Sharon O'Brien discusses of those who move from health to illness, routinely recording a time when life was better (271). His narrative is a through-story, a continuous "living with" that moves readers, not Al, from a before–*Spiral Cage* literacy to an after–*Spiral Cage* literacy. Or in their essay on disability and temporality in comics, Shoshana Magnet and Amanda Watson contend that by "refusing . . . to present only a coherent subject," comics repudiate ableism by also "'testify[ing] about, but . . . not reproduce[ing] trauma'" (Magnet and Watson quote Ann Cvetcovich n.p.). If Davison must create new neural pathways to physical mobility, his narrative requires readers to forge new literacy strategies that alter how they conventionally read, interpret, and (mis)judge impairment.[3] We have no choice but to collaborate with Davison by reading against literacy's anticipated grain as he also develops alternately.

Davison himself hoped *The Spiral Cage* would become "an educational tool" in schools, states McIlvenny (241). Not as a tool rehearsing the deterministic and pedantic nature of uplifting narratives about impairment in which a severely disabled child, medically doomed to an early death, surprisingly survives and thrives. Rather, argues McIlvenny, Davison's work redefines "disability as political oppression" (241). Children born with spina bifida, indeed, may be challenged by their own bodies. More difficult to overcome, however, are the unending taunts, ugly judgments, and downright despicable reactions they endure, argues McIlvenny (241). David Mitchell and Sharon Snyder suggest that readers trained by, or assimilated into, the culture of medicine and conventional literary plotting are obstacles for writers who wish to provide "other [narrative] options" limning their experiences of disability (Preface to *Narrative Prosthesis* xii). "In order to be disabled," they advance, "one must narrate one's disability for others in sweeping strokes or hushed private tones. Furthermore, such a narrative must inevitably show how subjects conquer disabilities or how they [the disabilities] eventually conquer subjects" (xii). *The Spiral Cage* speaks in no hushed tones, refuses to soften the hard edges of others' discrimination and cruelty against Al. "Comics are the thinking and not merely a format or forum for thinking," argues Michael Chaney in the introduction to his *Reading Lessons in Seeing*, significantly called "The Pupil, or the Instructional Unconscious of Comics" (5). However, reading *The Spiral Cage* through Davison's ruptures does not suspend identity, as Chaney argues, but rather assists us in forging Al's identity through the physical labor of reading the work. Davison first restrains, then retrains our cultured reading process—our expectations of the linearity of a bildungsroman or the assumed uplift of a disability narrative—through Al's versatile incorporation of corporeal limitations in an environment and culture built for the able bodied. Jared Gardner argues in his 2015 Graphic Medicine keynote "Beyond Metaphor" that the built-in repetition of comics iconography is a kind of OCD without an evident cure; comics, he concludes, are not about the conquest of disease, as our medical metaphors dictate, but about "testimony" as they work against the grain of medical ideology, medical narrative, and, I would add, reading practices. They replace Fricker's aforementioned testimonial injustice—disbelief in experiences voiced by the impaired—with their own images. Accepted definitions of impairment as deficiency can be altered, re-formed on the comics page. Davison's definitions are disciplinary reading strategies revising reader's approaches to ableist narratives. To reframe Chaney's argument, *The Spiral Cage* provides seeing lessons in reading.

That the reader is schooled through Davison's artistic repetitions to accept as normal the aberrant visual gymnastics of *The Spiral Cage* requires slow reading, repetitive reading, even somatic reading. What I call graphic genesis alludes first to how Al repudiates the limits of his bodily growth as assumed by the medical establishment. He progresses beyond such narrow parameters. Second, because the readers generate connections among initially seemingly incoherent image juxtapositions, they also advance beyond literacy's established parameters. Genesis references both the physicality of the body and the figurations of comics. Thierry Groensteen's concept of "braiding" usefully ropes the somatic and the graphic. Braiding occurs when iconic images reappear in strategic places as narrative links, falling under what he identifies as a general arthrology. Derived from the Greek "arthron" meaning articulation, arthrology is the study of joints and links in medicine (*System of Comics* 21), a particularly suitable approach to graphic narrative in which meaning is extracted not through prose but collectively across gutters, iconicity, and panel shapes. Arthrology asks readers to associate images among nonlinear panels. As Al develops the connections or sinews necessary for physical movement, so, too, do readers yoke the visual tendons of his comics with meaning. His myriad drawing styles of varied self-depictions require constant leaps of the imagination, so much so that reading for and with flexibility and mobility in a book about assumed paralysis becomes the norm. Disability as deficiency is turned on its head, wherein Davison illustrates how Rosemarie Garland-Thomson's concept of the "normate" in disability studies, the status quo's acceptance of a "normal" body, becomes untenable.[4] In this process of graphic genesis, readers arthrologize the many divisive experiences that compose Al's eventual self-confident persona. We assemble the parts into the entirety of Al, akin to McCloud's comics closure, in order to vitalize the text as Al invigorates himself from a baby once predicted as unviable.

Davison's graphic genesis is not a reading prosthesis as proposed by Mitchell and Snyder, as it refuses to mainstream impaired characters by erasing or assimilating disability's differences (*Narrative Prosthesis* 7).[5] Rather, as argued within recent essays on graphic pathography that revise reading practices so the impaired subject is no longer amenable (as "merely" a prop) to the narrative and its readers, Davison's narrative is prosthetically helpful, as outlined in the following scholarly theories about graphic pathography and in atypical (non-normate) graphic pathography itself. Consider a conceptual style that Chris Foss calls "literary autism" ("Reading in Pictures" 101). In a reading of Keiko Tobe's manga series *With the Light: Raising an Autistic Child*, Foss thoughtfully examines Tobe's emanata, onomatopoeia, "pictorial runes," and "indexical signs" that enlist several senses at once, and her frequent aspect-to-aspect transitions that set mood or establish location, according to McCloud, rather than advancing a plot (Foss 101). These comics strategies mimic a visually conceptual representation of an autistic view (Foss references Kazuko Shinohara and Yoshihiro Matsunaka 99). Shannon Walters also addresses a kind of Fossian literary autism when she questions the "neurotypical limits" of McCloud's notion of image and word closure, in which readers fill the gaps between panels, or complete familiar words or images, from partial representations (Walters 112). These oft-used comics elements unfortunately advance neurotypical approaches to reading graphic narrative. Walters suggests that prohibiting readers from filling gaps in a comic about an autistic subject may be another way for "part and whole" to operate (123). Mariah Crilley demonstrates how the typical, daily activities of walking or eating become "extraordinary feats" for characters suffering from Huntington's chorea in Steven Seagle and Teddy Kristiansen's *It's a Bird. . . .* This sense is conveyed by juxtaposing idiosyncratic images of Superman with the human character Steve, a protagonist genetically susceptible to Huntington's chorea. In Roland Burkart's *Twister*, about character Piedro paralyzed after fracturing a vertebra and learning to navigate by wheelchair, images of a happily whirling Piedro in his wheeled prosthetic sprawl across the page's white expanse. Uninhibited by panel reticulation, the layout reflects Piedro's capacious approach to life's sudden alterations, unwilling to be physically hobbled by a prosthesis. As critics argue, these graphic pathographies are not prosthetic narratives but rather visual strategies by which to cleave—both bridge and separate—ability and disability, nonimpairment and impairment.

Not Immediately Accessible: The Built Environment, Building Graphic Narrative's Environment

The built environment of cities, shopping malls, university campuses, and other public spaces remains largely inaccessible to many with physical impairment. A disabled body contrasts to what Tobin Siebers calls the "preferred social body" (85). Nonpreferred bodies whose access to such navigationally obstructing environments are impossible (impassable) only because they lack ramps, curb cuts, or automated doors. They thus are denied equal participation, exempted and restrained by elements beyond the physical limitations of their bodies. G. Thomas Couser claims that "a fundamental and crucial distinction is made between impairment, which is found in the body, and disability, which is located in the social response to, or cultural construction of, impairment" (*Signifying Bodies* 26). Reading is literacy's built environment. Those who are illiterate are excluded from participating in a host of daily, even necessary, activities. As Al conforms with great difficulty to an able-bodied world, so, too, do his visual arrangements impede our entrance into his graphic world as they deliberately chafe against our built (habitual) reading practices. Just as physical "constructions are built with social bodies in mind," argues Siebers about how space disciplines ability (124), Davison anchors the built (normate) reading process as an impediment to his autographic work. We are given no easy access to his comics, no literary curb cuts.

Those whose DNA restricts typical development—here Al's genetically engineered paralysis from the waist down—might grow otherwise, a metaphor for his eventual corporeal mobility. In my analysis of the "spiral" in the title *The Spiral Cage*, I allude to both a mode of circular reading and the DNA helix that contains the part of Al's genetic code resulting in the incomplete closure, in utero, of Al's spinal cord. That I have often mistyped the graphic pathography's title, substituting "spinal" for "spiral," attests intimate associations between the spine embedded in *spina* bifada and the spine embodied in our core as a stabilizing column. The confusion asserts itself constantly in my imagination. As an associative and able-bodied reader, I carelessly affiliate the terms, replacing the expected one with the other, not experienced by me, while Al's physical condition prohibits such complacency. As we work through his documented advances and retreats, we discard one reading to forge another in the built comics environment.

Taunted by peers, regarded as unintelligent by teachers, as asexual by strangers,[6] and generally cruelly diminished by those around him, Al navigates this built environment that expects those with spina bifida to grow (or devolve) into "your average vegetable" (Davison, *Spiral Cage*, 2003 8), an environment whose structures (physical, social, psychological) are produced with the normate in mind. Couser contends that "a particular condition or trait is regarded as a more or less transparent sign of the moral or spiritual status of an affected individual. One cost of this paradigm, then, even when it is not obviously prejudicial, is that it erases individual differences within the group marked as different. It makes a particular trait—say, deformity or blindness—the master status of all those who possess it, reducing their complex humanity to a single (usually visible) attribute" (*Signifying Bodies* 22). Others like Al adapt or find creative approaches to that which seems inaccessible, as does Al when he eventually admonishes the taunts of those who view him as crippled, damaged, asexual, and abnormal through a life of intellectual thought, mobility, cartooning, and, most importantly, love.[7]

On the comics page, Al's development from crutches to walking is not uninhibitedly forward moving nor is it stalled; he vacillates between the two both literally (or visually) and figuratively. When he is down, he is not necessarily depressed, although sometimes he is. When standing, he also can be down/depressed and so on. His state of being is not his state of mind. Or, as argued by Elisabeth El Refaie, "the spatial dimension of up and down becomes correlated from infancy onward with the experience of being upright and able to move about freely," promoting us "to talk about our state of happiness in terms of being "up(beat)" or "down(cast)" (El Refaie quotes Raymond Gibbs Jr. 1–2). Because Al has been unable to move about freely since infancy, the comics dehabituate us from the metaphors we live by.[8] Every panel depicting his successes might be followed by one depicting regression, physically or psychologically. But the alteration between the two is like muscle memory; two steps forward, a stumble, perhaps one step back. But as readers, we do not retreat enough to forget what advancing—otherwise, sideways—feels like. Overcoming structural obstacles and inequities in innovative ways demands that we, too, read sideways.

Queer studies, cultural studies, and comics studies have critiqued progress as unnecessarily attached to forward thinking and as future related. In *Feeling Backward: Loss and the Politics of Queer History*, Heather Love argues that queer stigmatization is freighted by a history (that which has come before) of loss, corporeal and psychological violence, discrimination, and despair.[9] These exceptions from the past, however, affirm queer existence in the future (3). In *The Queer Child, or Growing Sideways in the Twentieth Century*, Kathryn Bond Stockton argues that queer children might grow athwart of expected heterosexual orientation. Adults who manage—or more so obstruct—teens' natural curiosity direct young adults to seek answers in a roundabout way: a child instinctively leans *toward* understanding concepts and ideas beyond their ken, exhibiting a natural curiosity required for continued, intellectual growth. When authority figures refrain from offering explanations, when the child's path to comprehension is blocked, the youth arrives at requested definitions sideways, through other sources and means. Impediments to their intellectual curiosity prohibit upward, vertical growth, but growing sideways, or horizontally, claims Stockton, remains crucial to queer childhood (4).[10]

The Spiral Cage is built strategically to disrupt conventional acclimations of progression, as readers advance sideways or backward in order to move along (forward) in comprehension. The preface's final page, for example, consists of a series of identically sized panels that form a square border around a central image. Each panel presents a different stage of Al's development, from fetus to adult (fig. 1). The sequence, however, does not commence in the upper-left-hand corner, the starting point in Western literary practice, from which our eyes move "naturally" across the top of the page before plunging down the right-hand side in an assumed clockwise direction. In atypical reading fashion, the progressive sequence depicting Al as a growing fetus begins in the top right-hand corner, moves left across the top, then slides down the left-hand side, snaking counter clockwise around the framed central panel. As *The Spiral Cage* thwarts logical Western reading convention, the autographic's dis-chronology disaffectingly uncouples impairment from notions of awkward or wrong. El Refaie argues that "the arrangement of visual elements on a page is able to convey metaphorical meanings by drawing on our experience of our bodies in space" (7). An artist's experience of atypical proprioception because of impairment requires divergent images and metaphors that inform, in Al's case, how his body moves atypically through space. Faced with extrapolating meaning and logic from consistently different images and patterns that play with established literacy agreements, we adapt to change like Al, eventually normalizing continuous alterations to conformity. Davison's imagistic metalepses are surprising ocular reversions in service of graphic genesis.

Readers approach *The Spiral Cage* socially disciplined to stare at cartoon Al through any of the four types of "visual rhetoric" attributed to the visually conspicuous—to minority bodies—outlined by Garland-Thomson as the wondrous, the supercrip,[11] the sentimental, and the exotic ("The Politics of Staring" 59, 56). Readers may be unaware of how they see (or how we look, the subtitle of Garland-Thomson's study *On Staring*). Davison returns that ignorance to his readers. He makes natural the process of reading and rereading impairment. We do not know that we cannot read as we have been prescribed until we open *The Spiral Cage.*

I return us to Drew Leder's recessed body from the book's introduction, a healthy body that we may conveniently and consciously ignore—until we confront dysfunction through disease, disability, or pain. Born with spina bifida, Al's truncated mobility is naturally recessed in his own consciousness—he

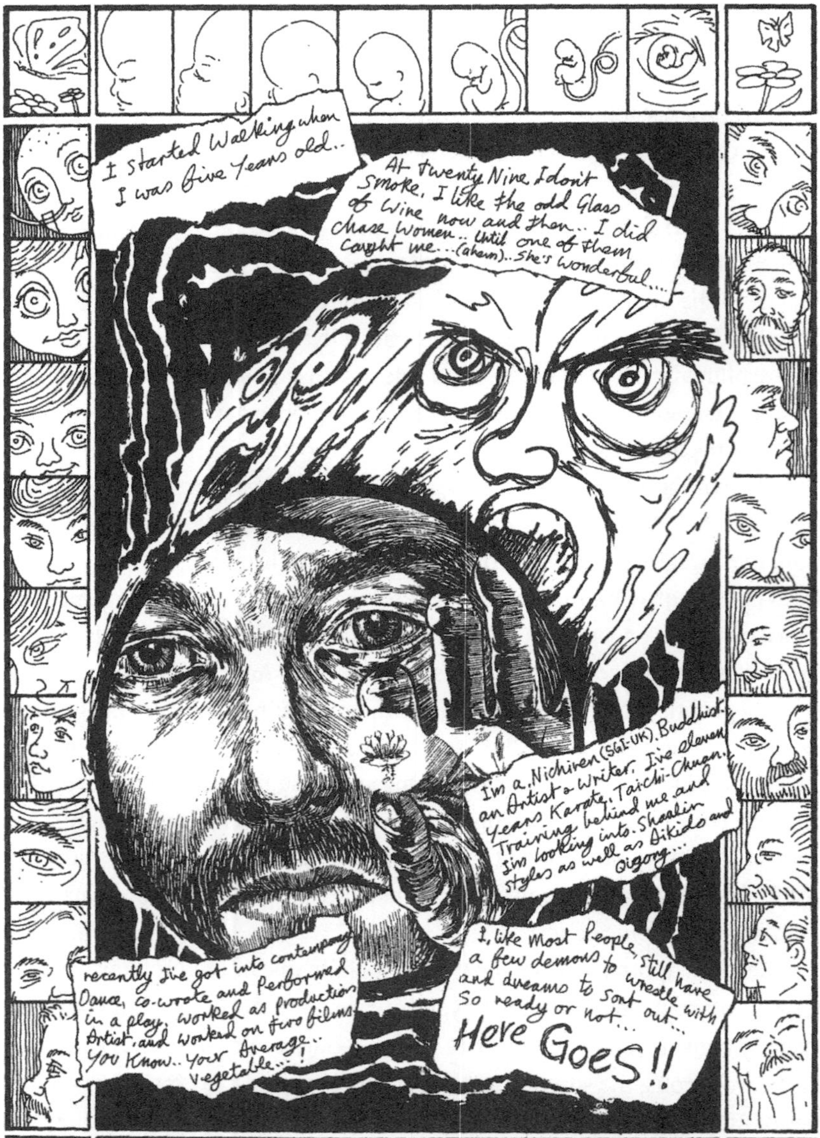
I started Walking when I was five Years old..
At twenty Nine I don't Smoke, I like the odd Glass of Wine now and then.. I did chase Women.. Until one of them caught me...(ahem)..She's wonderful....
I'm a Nichiren (SGI-UK) Buddhist, an Artist & Writer. I've eleven years Karate, Taichi-Chuan Training behind me and I'm looking into Shaolin styles as well as Aikido and Qigong...
recently I've got into contemporary Dance, co-wrote and Performed in a play, worked as production Artist, and worked on two films. You Know.. your Average.. vegetable...!
I, like Most People, still have a few demons to wrestle with and dreams to sort out... So ready or not...
Here Goes!!

Fig. 1 | Learning to read otherwise. Davison's *The Spiral Cage*, p. 8. Copyright © Al Davison / TAG!artworks, 2022.

knows nothing beyond the bodily capacities with which he was born—until he can no longer physically keep up with his older sister (although more mobile than her brother, she herself acclimates bodily to cerebral palsy). The disparaging words of other boys and men also continuously alert him to his corporeal difference; how "we" look affects Al's self-outlook, frustrating his psychological progression even as he defies clinical prognosis of his physical progression. Al eventually disciplines his body and mind, tutoring himself in somatic self-enhancement and self-confidence, to literally stand up to and stare back at his aggressors. In turn, we discipline ourselves to read *The Spiral Cage* sideways. Al incorporates elements of dysfunction into his life, accepting his originary body as natural.

Style, Ink, and Myth: Animating the Stationary, Dreaming Reality

Chaney's I-cons are graphic narrative's self-referential subjects (6). Davison's I-cons appear in a myriad of inconsistent drawing styles, from cross-hatched and detailed adult Al to scribbly baby Al, from a simple stick figure boyhood Al to an older photorealistic Al. Scholars discuss how various comics styles within a work allow authors' unique self-representation in autobiographic graphic narrative to self-depict at various nonchronological points in their lives and to signal characters' changing life circumstances. Flipping through Davison's comic, variation is clearly manifest, returning us to the hand as style—the "man" from "main" or hand in French—that controls the text's tone, instructs our reading, and redefines the so-called cage of disability appearing in the book's title. In her study of cartoonist Lynda Barry, Susan Kirtley lists some critics' interpretations of Barry's various drawing modes: "Busy boxes and askew lines reflect the scuffed look of childhood" or Barry's "cluttered and sinuous appearance of her ink lines . . . suggest the tension between the limitations of the format and Barry's efforts to expand what can be expressed within them" (41). Kirtley's own opinion about Barry's style argues that the artist's "raw, edgy aesthetic underscores the bumpy, jarring experience of childhood" (42). Hannah Miodrag finds that Charles Burns's articulated pen strokes in his *Black Hole* contribute to a menacing animation, as if the virus infecting the youth in his graphic pathography is quivering on the page, restless and intrusive and ultimately ominous (204–5).

"I always use the style to set the story," remarks Davison in an interview by Alex Fitch, inviting interpretive claims about the tone and shape of his design ("Panel Borders: *Doctor Who* and *The Spiral Cage*" podcast). Davison's predominant stylistic mode incorporates lots of ink: black backgrounds, heavy shading, extensive crosshatching, and ink spattering. The graphic pathography thus seems freighted with darkness. However, Davison's self-portraits are often more radiant and exuberant than not, his predominantly elated childhood visages full of hope and wonder. Scattered across the text, they are enlightening reminders of Al's indomitable spirit and that impairment in an able-bodied world can be a confining frame of mind—the reader's, but not Al's. Barring a systemic accounting that might find panels of Al's despair outnumbering those of ebullience, the narrative's general tone exudes happy vitality. In a three-page series near the beginning, infant Al, dozing in his crib, dreams that he is a boy with a mermaid's tail. Floating above his grounded, sleeping self, gleeful mermaid Al twists and turns effortlessly in the air. In the background, two nurses comment on his sleep patterns amid panels of Al's lithe and tumbling body, one remarking that the child does not yet need any medication, the other that "he giggles alot [*sic*] . . . he wakes up laughing" (22). Somersaulting in subsequent panels, Davison zooms in on Al's smiling, upturned face until the gamboling child suddenly starts to drop, flapping his arms with a sly grin on his face before disappearing with a downward "WWHEEEEE" into a visual image of a splash of water (22). We are trapped in an ideological prison of our own making if we pity Al as he spins and spirals out of the cage of his impairment to dance above us, light as air.

Davison's other graphic narratives gather dreams and references to mythology, often incorporating autobiographical materials about "ugly" humans who are disabled or disfigured, but only to render them incontrovertibly significant. His 1992 *The Minotaur's Tale* relates the myth from the viewpoint of the minotaur through a very loosely configured association: character Banshee possesses a grotesque face, waddles as does Al in *The Spiral Cage*, and only when he finally receives love from another can the narrator proclaim, "I pray that reading this, you will seek wisdom, dignity, and compassion within yourself, and in doing so attract these blessings from others" (n.p.). His 2009 *Hokusai: Demons—and Other Tales of the Fox Mother* vividly records some of his dream sequences in full color, sometimes in clear line style, other times by borrowing pictorial elements from Japanese manga and woodblock prints. In both, Davison clearly appreciates the naked human body in all of its idiosyncrasies, painting it with brushes, penning it in black ink, crafting it through soft washes and colored penciling. In her foreword to the collection *Disability in Comic Books and Graphic Narratives*, Garland-Thomson states that comics' "most distinct representational opportunity" is its use of hyperbole that assaults "the scale and order of what we take to be everyday reality" (xii). The "spectacle, irony, disorder, [and] distortion" that Garland-Thomson lists as elemental to comics ability to represent (xii) are routinized aspects of Al's life. It is not unusual, then, that Davison's I-cons meld reality and what readers view as myth, fragments of his own fantastic life.

The Materiality of the Book: Disintegration and Regeneration

In this section, I explore corporality through materiality in the evolution, over decades, of *The Spiral Cage*'s materiality from floppy magazine to more substantial softcover publication. My reading suggests another avenue by which to think about graphic genesis as a form of regeneration, a becoming. The graphic narrative emerged from Davison's "visual diary," kept from 1984 to 1988 (Fitch's podcast). The 1988 Renegade version (Long Beach, California), titled *The Spiral Cage: Diary of an Astral Gypsy*, is thin at a mere 56 pages, more like what we imagine when we say "comics"; given this insubstantiality, it is not surprising that the original binding disintegrated. It was pulled from the shelves and replaced with the 1994 expanded 112-page Titan (London) version, hefty with the weight of added materials and organized now by chapters.[12] In 2003, it was reissued by Active Images (Los Angeles, California), including even more material, bringing the page count to 140. The successive versions interest me on two fronts: how they "grew up" from comics to graphic narratives, and their materiality in relation to the body. They reflect Al's various incarnations, or his graphic (comics and bodily) genesis, from an initial fragility to a self-possessed solidity.

In the recent past, scholars have valued graphic narrative as a medium worthy of a sophisticated (adult) audience by pointing to its complex themes and intricate word-image composition, those *affordances* of this multimodal medium. Current comics scholarship has grown out of—or beyond—this defensive posture, assuming comics' explicit value among academic and non-academic readers alike without needing to continuously argue for it. Interestingly, the successive publications of *The Spiral Cage* reflect similar iterations by which we come to appreciate Al's corporeality. Davison re-visions capability to wrest impairment (self-possessed embodiment) from disability (cultural obstruction) until he no longer needs to substantiate it. The value of such honing—falling and standing—is akin to the Buddhist ritual of polishing one's mirror to affirm oneself, as Al practices himself (Davison, *Spiral Cage* 123). He eventually turns the mirror toward his readers as if asking, what do *you* see in yourself that shapes how you *see* me? Graphic pathographies "move the focus from *looking at* a sick body to *looking out* at the reader," argues Jodi Cressman, in order to fashion an ethical "embodied witness who sees and is seen" (emphasis in original 23).

Many of what we now consider seminal graphic narratives were once serialized comics, including Art Spiegelman's *Maus I* and *II*, Harvey Pekar's *American Splendor*, and Alan Moore and Dave Gibbons's *Watchmen*. Many early serialized autographies emerged from the so-called juvenility of low-brow comics into the maturity of high-brow graphic narrative, a popular argument about their trajectory that counters the charge that comics are unsuitable material for scholarly study and classroom pedagogy.[13] Repeatedly, comics scholars have had to prove the medium's worth amid resistant expert and lay opinions. Roger Sabin commences his history of the medium, *Comics, Comix and Graphic Novels: A History of Comic Art*, by explaining that even though comics "have smuggled their way into art books," they reside there "as an aside, a digression, to demonstrate the inspiration for the 'proper' art that constitutes the bulk of the book" (1).[14] According to Bart Beaty, pigeonholing "hybrid art forms" (comics text-and-image combinations) as literature for youth subsequently permits an overlooking of their aesthetic qualities (21). He exemplifies that Spiegelman's *Maus* takes us from the "low" (of rats and mice) to high art (124). Comics found solid footing in the early twenty-first century, evidenced by the rising number of journals publishing comics scholarship; the rapidly growing number of monographs on comics themes and artists, especially by Penn State University Press, the University Press of Mississippi, and The Ohio State University Press; a rise in college courses focused specifically on comics; an expanding number of panels at major domestic conference venues featuring comics criticism as well as numerous international comics-only themed conferences; and, finally, the change in nomenclature from comics to graphic narrative (and graphic novels), suggesting a rise from comics' association with youth to a medium capturing and captivating wider audiences, even though adults have always participated, for over a century, in reading comics, comic strips, and cartoons.

The 2003 Active Image publication of *The Spiral Cage* includes an introduction by Alan Moore, whose literary presence auspiciously tethers aspects of superhero comics to graphic narrative, an association that seems to rehearse the comics-for-kids argument until he explodes it. Moore began his career writing for DC before authoring the initially serialized anti-superhero *Watchmen* (story by Moore, artwork by Gibbons) that propelled him into the limelight. If comics scholars have marked an advancement from superhero comics to graphic narrative—I note my own distinguishing language here such as "advancing" and "rising"—Moore has risen, then, from the so-called depths of comics for children to the heights of mature graphic texts for adults. But Moore's distinction in his introduction to *The Spiral Cage* between "juvenile superhero comics" with its "rigid perimeters [*sic*]" (3, 4) is not one of childish literature versus a sophisticated adult medium. Moore simply suggests that the comic book audience is changing while scholars inflect *change* by introducing comics' rich academic potential to the academy. Locating the "all-too-human" in Davison's work, not "the unreachably superhuman," Moore reverses assumed directional moves—from youthful comics to serious adult graphic narrative—embraced by scholars in the field (4). To bring Davison's *The Spiral Cage* down to earth is not to degrade it. Rather, Moore elevates the superhero to the unreachable, rendering Davison's graphic narrative the normative, the all-too-human. Davison himself is no superhero but self-values despite, or even because, his body's genetic inclination is to follow a different somatic path.

If the first Renegade edition's binding, or the book's spine, resonates with the spinal differences of Davison's spina bifida, then the material book's development into a studier graphic narrative reflects Davison's own physical augmentation otherwise (becoming a karate expert, for example) in concert with establishing and fortifying a healthy psychological state. The materiality of the book—heftier, stronger, more durable—mimics the growing corporeal and mental vitality and tenacity of its artist.[15] Each new version develops by the addition of pages, expanding the narrative sideways. A comic is, indeed, tethered to and supported by its binding, its spine. For Groensteen, arthrology, discussed earlier, is comics' figurative corporeal feature of panel layouts, motifs, or images woven together by the reader. Arthrology is parts in service to a conceptual whole. Movement, specifically readers' eye movement, in *The Spiral Cage* must stray from its learned groove for us to acknowledge that "the positioning of the frames . . . adjust to each other on the model of fractured bones knitting together, organizing themselves into the page layout" (Groensteen, *Comics and Narration* 34). Davison's many panels are in seeming disarray, as if a leg is bent in a so-called wrong direction, but eventually cohere through numerous close readings. The leg bone really is connected to the ankle bone, the text suggests. If Al's spina bifida is an exposed spine at birth that paralyzes his legs, the arthrology of his book is carefully stitched into the panels, united by an active reading process.[16]

In our hands, we hold and behold Davison's hand-drawn work of embodiment. Davison's panels are free to wander among what Groensteen argues is comics' "innovative current characterized by a poetics of reticence, ambiguity, and indeterminacy . . . eschewing the kind of relationships that are immediately decodable in terms of narrative logic and meaning" (*Comics and Narration* 30). In an age no longer subjected to what Groensteen calls classic comics' submission to "the imperialism of narration," Davison's meandering visual telling refuses to be disciplined by a linear, progressive form as Al refuses bodily compliance to expected prognosis and development. His graphic genesis is both an autobiographical strategy and a reading exercise.

Walking in Al's World: A Conclusion

Sarah Brophy and Janice Hladki argue that in visual autobiography, the works "embed negation" or "refuse affective connectivity even as they *demand* it" (emphasis in original 244). That is, the unimpaired cannot fully comprehend how the (concretely and socially) built environment impedes mobility of the impaired or how culture's homogenizing norms invite "ugly" looks directed toward impaired subjects. Yet if Patrick Devlieger and proponents of DISABILITY MUNDUS propose "world perspectives on disability" (13) in which impairment is both a world of its own and of the world, then an unimpaired circulation within the *mundus* includes—ultimately demands—connectivity with those subjects who are impaired.[17] Davison's *The Spiral Cage* draws against the testimonial injustice about minority bodies, argued by Barnes. Reeducated in literacy techniques about this minority body, readers of Davison's *The Spiral Cage* adjust to an initial inability to read before acclimating to the comics' built environment to walk, even if marginally, in Al's world.

Zach Whalen, Chris Foss, and Jonathan Gray claim, "Disability . . . [is] one of the most fundamental and increasingly significant components to human identity" (2). In the next chapter, women's bodies specifically are viewed as sites of identity creation through standards of (white) beauty, body size and weight, and economic class, all of which contribute to overlapping assumptions about women "fighting" breast cancer and other diseases. Character Al's refusal to submit to given identities is accepted as valuable, but what is deemed "good" or "bad" for ill women—or, more pointedly, which women are considered "good" and which "bad"—means confronting an altogether different standard.

Chapter 2

Facing Cancer, the Face of Cancer

Beauty, Health, and Affect in Marchetto's *Cancer Vixen* and *Ann Tenna*

Feminist theorists have turned to the material body as "a site for understanding the interrelationships of identities, subjectivities, and health," proclaims Courtney Donovan (239). No longer merely a discursive, post-structural construction, the body is a physical reality in which pain and disease are embodied. And because each woman's bodily experiences are unique, they provide unlimited sources of visual knowledge about illness.[1] In this chapter, the myriad of lived sensations informing graphic pathography exceeds the boundaries of medicine's image archive. Graphic pathography individualizes experiences, as each ill or traumatized body "falls" into new sensations, a term suggested by Einat Avrahami in her study of autobiographies by subjects encountering terminal illness. No medical archive can accommodate this fall into disease and its enormous range of unique self-representative feelings. An individual's pathography is an innovatively imagined life on the page that contributes to and defamiliarizes us from an archive of clinical imagining. The history of medicine is also a chronicle of images through which bodies have been construed and subsequently confined, disciplined, and catalogued under a clinical gaze.[2] Medical registers that surveilled, documented, and circulated a narrow range of (white) bodies experiencing disease advanced this specific pathological embodiment to a wide range of other bodies, often in concert with social expectations about gender. In two graphic pathographies by the *New York Times* best-selling author Marisa Acocella Marchetto, *Cancer Vixen: A True Story* and *Ann Tenna*, the bodies of the women characters who fall into cancer and near-death, respectively, are platforms for discussing medi-

cal assumptions circumscribing women and health.[3] They remind us of tenacious scripts about how to psychologically wage war against cancer and about persistent cultural portraits of what constitutes feminine beauty, in sickness and in health. Both graphic narratives reflect rebellious white women who craft their own views of cancer and womanhood against conventional scripts.

This chapter focuses on images by women about their (ill or impaired) bodies with specific reference to pliable cartoon faces as conduits of emotion. Taking up the ubiquitous phrase "facing cancer," I first unpack the term "face" as both noun and verb, referencing a gendered history that has instructed women how to *face* cancer with uncompromising will, becoming the expected invulnerable *face* of cancer. Marchetto's characters generate other attitudes (faces) of cancer (*Cancer Vixen*) and wounding (*Ann Tenna*) that thwart medically promoted constructions of women, health, and beauty. Because both graphic pathographies also refer to women's bodies as sites of identity, especially cross-textually and in relation to other women, they incite productive, intersecting dialogues about "bad" diseases and "good" women. Relying on Sarah Ahmed's definition of affect, I then demonstrate how such accepted cultural scripts about women and illness circulate as capital among and beyond the affected/afflicted characters.

Narrative Synopses

In her graphic memoir *Cancer Vixen: A True Story*, author and artist Marchetto illustrates her year-long encounter with breast cancer, from diagnosis to chemotherapy to remission. She informs us of her successful cartooning career before the devastating discovery of a lump in her breast: "I was the *New York Times's* first cartoonist ever with 'The Strip,' which ran every other Sunday in the 'Styles' section," she rightfully boasts (*Cancer Vixen* 17). She lives a free-spirited life of fashion, good food, and wine and revels in feeling and looking great. In her opinion, she has had far too many bad boyfriends at the age of forty-three—until her engagement to Silvano, a successful, attractive (both in looks and pocketbook) restaurateur. The narrative begins with Marisa's cancer diagnosis three weeks before her wedding.

Marisa manages her illness through meticulous attention to her looks—her face—and by leveraging an attitudinal levity. Not to be overlooked, however, is her fiancé's substantial financial contributions to her care, including providing health insurance when Marisa's lapses. Marisa's cancer itself possesses a literal face: it appears as a personified cartoon cell, in a striking shade of green, giving the finger to Marisa from its position in a petri dish. Marisa returns the emotional impulse in kind: through a spirited, humorous, unrepentant, and literally colorful refusal to let cancer kick her ass. Throughout her chemotherapy and radiation treatments, Marisa retains her glamorous looks and active lifestyle despite how cancer treatments render her ill, ravage her skin, her weight, and her moods. A fleet of expensive shoes, for example, one outrageously fashionable pair for each of seven chemotherapy treatments, boosts (or boots) her self-confidence. From bejeweled Giuseppe Zanotti heeled mules (159) to embroidered magenta Casadei Faux Crocs (167), Marisa is ultra-fashionable even when she feels ultra-sick. Sassy and sexy in spite of cancer, she is the good (white) woman because she fights cancer in a bad (read: ferocious) way.

In her subsequent futuristic graphic narrative *Ann Tenna*, the fictional, attractive, and haughty fashionista Ann—suddenly rendered unsightly after surviving a near-fatal car accident—is a "bad" white woman in her repugnant desire to bring low all those women she deems more beautiful than she. Her popular blog Eye Mauler successfully and dispassionately "mauls" or destroys other women's public reputations. According to competitive Ann, compassion is for the dull and unsuccessful. That the accident involved her chauffeured SUV colliding with a garbage truck invites a delightful metaphor riffing on this "trash-talking gossip columnist" who suffers from a brain injury and hypoxia "from [literal] garbage in her mouth" (n.p.). From the accident forward, this ruthless, vindictive protagonist spends much of the graphic narrative as a terrifyingly ugly, but healing patient, first facially, later attitudinally. Her shuttered black eye, blistered lips, and bleeding nose of her blue, blighted face are the outward manifestations of her currently ugly personality. Ann fortunately possesses a "higher self," a "super consciousness" known as SuperAnn, who teaches "lower" Ann lessons in humility, morality, and kindness, or in "cleaning up some serious karma" (n.p.) (fig. 2).[4] SuperAnn had banished Ann to earth, or "damnesia" (n.p.), for her malicious conceit, only permitted to return to a better place—and more beautiful face—after she cleans up her act. Ann's vindictive and petty earthly self knows better than to act as she does in her current lowly place on earth but stubbornly refuses to act on that impulse because greed and narcissism bring

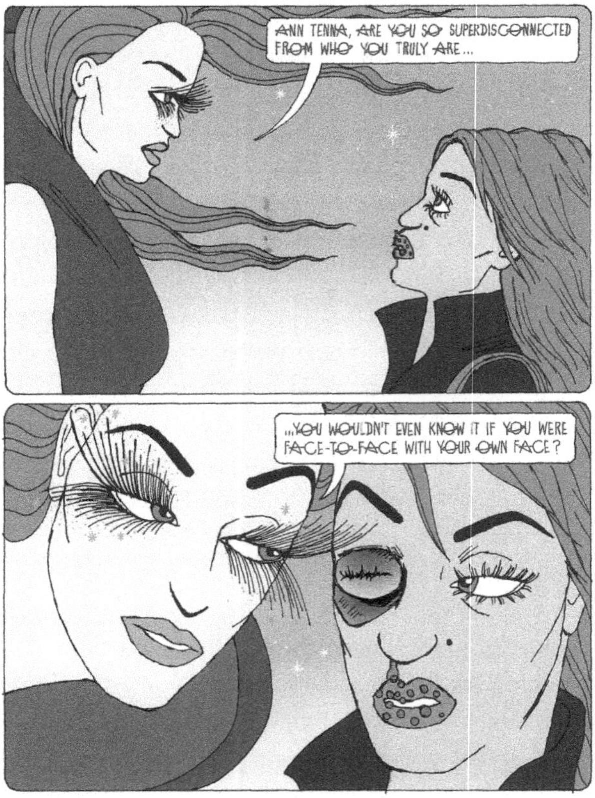
ANN TENNA, ARE YOU SO SUPERDISCONNECTED FROM WHO YOU TRULY ARE...
...YOU WOULDN'T EVEN KNOW IT IF YOU WERE FACE-TO-FACE WITH YOUR OWN FACE?

Fig. 2 | After her accident, Ann meets SuperAnn, her higher, better self. From Marisa Acocella Marchetto, *Ann Tenna*, 2015, n.p. Courtesy of Marisa Marchetto.

her wealth and admiration. Only after her exterior beauty is damaged can she experience deep humility to repair her inner self. Experiences of being brought low, humbled and humiliated by ugliness and remorse, eventually lead to her self-enlightenment. She is invited to literally go high, to live up to her appellation SuperAnn and reclaim her space in the celestial world from whence she has fallen.

The Many Faces of Cancer

"Face" can operate as both a noun and a verb, iterated above. As a noun in Marchetto's graphic pathographies, Marisa and Ann possess beautiful literal faces, the former miraculously sustained throughout her cancer ordeal, the latter able to reclaim her good looks only after reforming her petulant demeanor. As a verb in the phrase "to face cancer," it advances an attitude toward the disease, from stoicism to surrender. The former disposition has been elevated over the latter, intoning that those who "face" cancer with internal determination and tenacity are considered more courageous ("good") than those approaching the daunting disease with weakness and resignation ("bad"). One evaluation confers admiration on the afflicted, the other chastises. Consider the paratextual marketing materials of two exemplary graphic pathographies about cancer. Prose on the back cover of Stan Mack's *Janet and Me: An Illustrated Story of Love and Loss* states that the work delineates "a [white] woman who *faced* her cancer the same way she lived her life, with guts and charm" (emphasis added). The back cover of *Our Cancer Year*, authored by Harvey Pekar and Joyce Brabner, illustrated by Frank Stack, states that comics avatar Harvey confronts cancer "kicking, screaming, and complaining all the way." What implications does this rationing of a set of tropes or images hold for Marchetto's women protagonists? Graphic pathography attends to narratives that accuse or recuse in order to explore cancer's many faces.

If the history of medicine is a history of constraining metaphors, suggested by Susan Sontag, it also contains a history of medical images by which patients accord themselves. Sontag's *Illness as Metaphor and AIDS and Its Metaphors*, originally published in 1978 and 1989 respectively, and extremely influential in cultural studies and the medical humanities, elucidated a cultural approach to managing "good" and "bad" (predominantly white) subjects of disease. Social perceptions of cancer or AIDS validated some patients over others—permitted some more sympathy than others—depending on the origins of the affliction. Smokers with lung cancer, for example, received less compassion than those whose cancer sources remained ambiguous, perhaps environmental. The latter attitude shifted blame from individual (smoking) actors—well-informed of the dangers of nicotine but nonetheless actively contributing to their own demise—to passive victims unknowingly arrested by toxic, airborne chemicals circulating invisibly in the air, water, or engineered food on the table. More recently, breast cancer victims have been renamed "survivors," according to Samantha King (107), in which adopting a positive or "right" frame of mind that channels upbeat optimism peddles society's positive thinking as cure (King quotes Barbara Ehrenrich 103). In the realm of cancer scholarship, Gayle Sulik alludes to this as "pink ribbon ideology," a mentality that shifts the responsibility of fighting cancer from the medical realm to the individual. In that shift, she who succumbs to cancer might be regarded as an individual who did not try hard enough to live positively, hence allowing society to censure (per Sontag) the already victimized subject. Emily Waples calls cancer success stories tales of "triumph" in contrast to those of "declension" (159). She notes that victory over death suggests that living is a choice grounded in personal achievement (159). Those who die chose not to battle hard enough for life. Meanwhile, Diane Price Herndl poses trenchant questions, relevant to this study, about the nature of cancer autobiographies that generally "paint a positive picture of recovery and healing: but are such narratives un-problematically true? What are their political consequences? In what ways do the body, its inadequacies, and its fragmentation become part of a new narrative identity?" (222).

Or more importantly, I ask, whose narrative identity? Implications about Sontag's metaphors as gendered or, significantly here as racialized, remain dormant, argues Keith Wailoo. His *How Cancer Crossed the Color Line* considers what perceptions about race and cancer in the first half of the twentieth century shaped who received care and of what quality. "Cancer awareness was far more than a health campaign; it was an expertly targeted social ideology" attending predominantly to white women. Theories of "racial biology or genetic difference" shaped narratives of white women's natural fragility against black women's assumed fortitude (5). Hence, robust medical attention to white women suffering from breast, uterine, ovarian, or vaginal cancer met several nefarious goals. It promulgated an incontrovertible narrative to safeguard white babies. It hid black women's cancerous afflictions, as their absence from the cancer wards reinforced damaging ideology about black women's so-called natural resistance to disease. Beneath these proclamations that were eventually enfolded seamlessly into the wider health care realm and refracted back to society lay the acceptance of cancer as a "white disease" (3). Cancer's *face* throughout the first half of the twentieth century was a white one (2). Whose cancer face we encounter in graphic pathography is thus unsurprising. Marisa, a white upper-middle-class woman whose health insurance is paid for by her wealthy fiancé, reflects only one of cancer's many faces. Persistent questions in the twenty-first century about why other, nonwhite faces get attached to inequitable access to, say, COVID-19 vaccinations and subsequent necessary hospitalizations, or are regarded as harbingers of the coronavirus itself (such as Asians and Asian North Americans) are addressed specifically in the book's coda.

Health care providers also *face* cancer in curative and palliative regimes for their patients. What faces do they project to their patients? How are they shaped and what do they convey? What face do patients return? Students in Kimberly Myers's 2012 course "Pathography: Reading and Writing the Patient," designed for fourth-year medical students at Penn State University's College of Medicine, were assigned to read nurses' visages in *Cancer Vixen*. Their strange "hyper-wide smiles and hyper-open eyes" indicate a possible "avoidance" of imparting bad news, Meyers's students claim (94). In "The Many Fictions of Illness," Antonio Ferraro argues that Brian Fies, creator of *Mom's Cancer*, depicts similar facial contortions in a physician's "jack-o-lantern" smile, the "ghoulish grin" revealing neatly arrayed teeth that take up nearly a third of the panel (241). Beneath the grinning veneer lies a message beyond the doctor's professed "You're doing just fine" that comics avatar Bill, his siblings, and his mother decode as sinister (Fies quoted by Ferraro 242); that is, the conscientiously managed expressions exhibited by health care providers that intend to relay comfort "don't put patients at ease" (94). For Judy Segal, "illness narratives not only document and catalogue experience, they also reflect and reinscribe a hierarchy of values [I would add expressions] for such experience: humour is good; despair is bad; surviving is noble; dying, by implication, is not" (Segal quoted by Ferraro 230).

Amid the rise of literature and medicine, a spate of books in cultural and literary studies in the decade from the early 1990s to the early 2000s explored how women's bodies appeared in medicine. Their contributions to the medical humanities critiqued longstanding medical and cultural views that erroneously promoted, for example, women's reproductive systems as passive players in fertilization (eggs were regarded as mere receptacles for active, egg-seeking sperm, as outlined by Emily Martin's *The Woman in the Body: A Cultural Analysis of Reproduction*) or characterized ill women as already invalid subjects (in Diane Price Herndl's *Invalid Women: Figuring Feminine Illness in American Fiction and Culture, 1840–1940*.) The studies mapped how tropes constructing women's so-called natural frailty informed scientific discourse that returned these discourses to culture, influencing women's self-descriptions.[5] Images impact and might persist destructively unless they are interrupted or reconstrued. At the same time, Sander Gilman was inquiring, "What can explain the anxiety of historians of medicine about the use of visual images?" (*Picturing Health and Illness* 9).[6] His history of medical illustrations, *Picturing Health and Illness*, is an academic exercise to answer his own query. Nineteenth-century clinical photography, for example, once participated in archiving the "look" of madness, erroneously attributing certain physiological features to insanity. The prescribing images both established insanity and were used to visually root it out among specific, lower-class populations.[7] Especially germane are references to women post–World War II who boldly intervened in medicine's staid depiction of women afflicted by disease, claims Ludmilla Jordanova. She refers to now-deceased breast cancer patient Jo Spence, who used her nude body, here through "autobiographical photography," to comment on her unsettling experiences under "orthodox medicine" ("Medicine and the Visual Arts" 55). Later, such women image pioneers are joined by disability activists who employ "public imagery" to destabilize its historic, negative "look" of disability that have shaped damaging self-representations of the impaired self (41).

Herein lie not only political results of art against orthodox medicine but also therapeutic promises of self-representative art intersecting with medicine. Avrahami argues that each individual's encounter and subsequent rendezvous with disease (or mental illness, or impairment) and any side effects from curative practices like the use of chemotherapy (or, in the past, madness's cure by lobotomy) progress beyond designations provided by medicine.[8] The real, or specific experiences of each patient, defies general, accepted clinical discourse and imaging about cancer, disease, and madness. Every graphic pathography attaches individual significance to each illustrated stage of living before, during, and after disease. In many ways, graphic pathography rebukes the afterlives of images.[9]

If Marchetto's graphic narratives interrupt a history of medical images, what do Marisa and Ann's self-representations as a cancer patient and amid disfiguration tell us about women and the body, women and cancer, facing cancer, and the face of cancer? By abandoning her judgment of other women, in accepting them as allies not rivals, we approve of Ann's "good" attitudinal change at the graphic narrative's conclusion that warrants her elevation to SuperAnn, moral and beautiful. Meanwhile, Marisa turns to envy, negative appraisal, and an overweening ego to overcome cancer, "bad" qualities that persist beyond remission. Is Marisa a good subject of a bad disease, or is Ann? When are women's learned practices of competing with other women or practicing self-inflation to combat social belittlement no longer necessary? My comparative reading of *Cancer Vixen* and *Ann Tenna* addresses these inquiries.

Women Visible to Each Other

In Audre Lorde's *The Cancer Journals*, penned before and after her mastectomy, she argues for "every woman to live a considered life" (57) so women can become "less and less willing . . . to passively accept external and destructive controls over our lives and our identities" (58). External controls allude to environmental toxins that often produce cancer, while controls over identities include clinical and social narratives and images that narrowly bind women's individual encounters to their embodiment of cancer. Lorde advocates for prevention, such as environmental detoxification (71), but before any of that, she asserts, "women with mastectomies must become visible to each other" (61). Encounters with disease in Marchetto's graphic narratives allow ill women to be made visible to each other, but in vastly different ways than Lorde may have imagined and to various results. Paired, the narratives represent a beauty-and-the-beast trajectory. Described earlier, Marisa practices daily self-indulgence in what society might deem an ugly vanity. Meanwhile, in wearing her battered face for months, Ann eventually cultivates a compassionate personality. In short, Marisa uses vanity to fight illness; Ann employs illness to fight vanity, the latter a seeming corrective to the former. How they each approach cancer and conceit, however, transcends collective, prescriptive approaches to embodying cancer and claiming inner beauty.

Marisa and Ann willingly participate in what Susan Bordo finds to be a "complexly and densely institutionalized *system* of values and practices within which girls and women—and, increasingly, men and boys—come to believe that they are nothing (and are frequently treated as nothing) unless they are trim, tight, lineless, bulgeless, and sagless" (emphasis in original 32). Persistent medical scripts about women work closely with those about feminine beauty. Women's expected adherence to culturally constructed representations of "attractive" bodies speaks to an equally constructed notion of self-control, or lack thereof (Bordo 58). Those who let go, who tolerate wrinkles and fleshly drooping, especially if they are not ill, are judged as lazy, sloppy, out of bodily and psychological self-regulation. Gazed at and judged long enough, women thus become their own overseers (see Bordo on Foucault 27). That which Marisa and Ann exude and circulate—a superior kind of beauty achieved only through self-control, so coerced to believe—affects their convalescence as well as negatively influences those who assist or compete against them in a circulation of affect.

On Affect

While affect in prose narratives has enjoyed scholarly popularity recently, its value in demonstrating how graphic narrative visualizes feelings on the page has been left unexplored. In *The Cultural Politics of Emotion*, Sara Ahmed argues that emotions work as a form of capital. They gain value as they circulate, and hence we can capitalize on emotions. Cancer has emotion, suggests Ahmed, not in the sense that a cancer cell or cancerous tumor "feels," but in that it produces affect in human beings as part of a larger distribution system of feelings about or toward cancer. Cancer does not, in fact, possess emotion but rather circulates it. No object or person "has" emotion; rather, emotions are economies that circulate between bodies, creating affective values. Extrapolating from Ahmed, cancer therefore does something. The term "cancer" evokes a flood of emotion for those who have been diagnosed, those never inflicted by it, for survivors in permanent remission, and for witnesses of its effects on friends and family.

Affect as a circulating entity for Ahmed yields public and political statements of, broadly, nationality, belonging, and inclusion. Counter to prediction, however, the negativity bound up in exclusion—those refused admittance into accepted realms replete with valuable cultural capital—produces conditions of inclusion. Affiliation produced through exclusion circulates as a positive form of affirmation. Jasbir Puar explores this configuration among gay Americans who understand the indignity and pain of discrimination, yet similarly victimized Middle Easterners after 9/11 by considering them terrorists. The once-excluded gay and lesbian population finds inclusion in homonationalism by ostracizing a group deemed nonnational and, in the latter's seemingly terrorist propensities, anti-nationalist, anti-American.[10] Collective adversity promotes affirmation. For Sianne Ngai, emotions that might invite exclusion are "ugly feelings."[11] Irritation, envy, anxiety, or disgust, she asserts, are negative emotions not only because they can be unsightly (an arrogant face can be an unattractive one) but also because they involve being or feeling "against" rather than toward (11). This negativity encapsulates a "suspended energy" driven by disenfranchisement (12).[12]

Social affect possesses an influencing ambiance that promotes the "good" desire to combat cancer amid a "bad" competition among women whose tenacious adherence to impossible beauty standards, even when ill, drive ugly feelings of jealousy. When protagonist Marisa's "fabulous life" is interrupted by cancer (*Cancer Vixen* 1)—which Martha Stoddard Holmes views as Marisa's shallow "cosmetic challenge" (Holmes 158)—she hopes to prohibit the so-called ugly cancer inside her body from affecting her beautiful exterior. This personal battle is staged on her body, against cancer, and often against others. Jealousy, for example, is illustrated as an actual fight between a sinewy red-hued (angry) Marisa with a trash can over her head, to suggest her bad behavior, and an anorexic blonde rival who wonders why she and all of her model friends never got hit on by Marisa's fiancé Silvano. Marisa as a monster red with jealousy literally rips off the blonde rival woman's head by her ponytail (56) (fig. 3). Her explosive anger illustrates how she also will encounter, head-on, her arresting chemotherapy. Fighting cancer in *Cancer Vixen* makes everybody unbecoming.

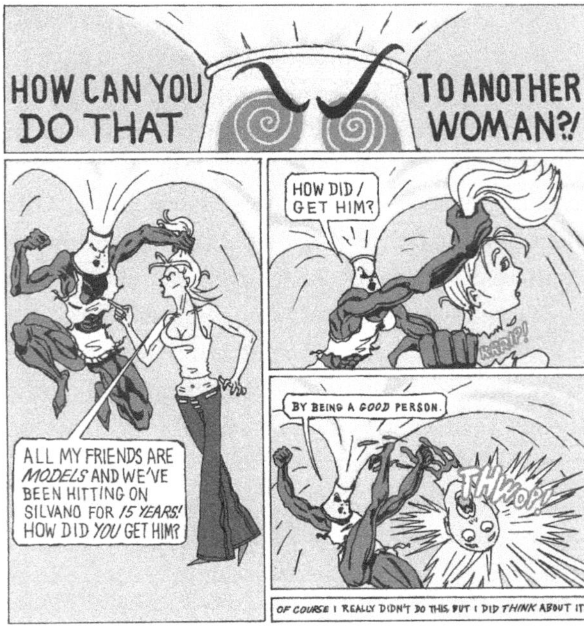
HOW CAN YOU DO THAT TO ANOTHER WOMAN?!
ALL MY FRIENDS ARE MODELS AND WE'VE BEEN HITTING ON SILVANO FOR 15 YEARS! HOW DID YOU GET HIM?
HOW DID I GET HIM?
BY BEING A GOOD PERSON.
THWOP!
OF COURSE I REALLY DIDN'T DO THIS, BUT I DID THINK ABOUT IT.

Fig. 3 | Marisa as a red monster of jealousy. From Marisa Acocella Marchetto, *Cancer Vixen*, 2006, p. 56. Courtesy of Marisa Acocella Marchetto.

An unflattering Ann in *Ann Tenna* takes advantage of her first-world white privilege and wealth to unconscionable ends. Ann's charitable contribution to women in Afghanistan, "denied their fundamental human rights" (n.p.), will be a special product from her own brand. Ann announces this, to much fanfare, amid a live assembled crowd of a women's worldwide coalition, as well as to the largest TV audience of her career. "The one thing that always made me feel powerful" is lipstick (n.p.), Ann's untenable first-world panacea to third-world challenges. She is immediately shouted down for her covert racism by a contingent of women watchdogs, Ann's frenemies in the audience, who loudly inform the crowd that Ann smuggled into Afghanistan expired "Velveeta Orange lipstick" from her father's pharmaceutical company (n.p.). Ann's more overt racism arises in the treatment of her chauffeur Lorna, a Peruvian Incan mystic who spent six months in prison after being convicted of grand theft, the latter a fact by which Ann blackmails her. As long as Lorna remains afraid and thus invaluably subservient, Ann will secure her background from the public eye. After Ann's turn of heart, an about-face at the graphic narrative's conclusion, she literally digs Lorna out of the trash. Marchetto winkingly employs a paradigm akin to the trope of the magical negro: Marchetto deems Lorna the brown woman who saves the white woman from herself.

The graphic pathographies work synergistically as elements of Ann's and Marisa's facial features and reactions to encroaching dis-ease mirror each other. Before the accident, Ann is a redheaded beauty; post-crash, her gray-purple pallor channels the walking dead. Yet their illustrated visages are remarkably similar, from their facial moles to a comparable tilting of the head, cast of the eyes, and analogous rendering of their noses and mouths. One might think that, other than their vastly different shades of hair, these are the same character. Such congruencies invite me to consider the 2015 *Ann Tenna* as an illustrated response, even a corrective, to the 2009 *Cancer Vixen*. The latter recuperates the former. Paired, the narratives represent a kind of beauty-and-the-beast trajectory. Despite the substantial correlation between them, however, Ann breaks from selfish indulgence while Marisa is trapped in social narratives defining beauty and their maliciously circulating affects. That a rehabilitated selfless, even upgraded, Ann follows closely on the heels of a self-centered Marisa suggests that the latter is an enhanced version of the former, promoting a recuperative dialogue between the graphic pathographies.

The circulation of affect in *Cancer Vixen*'s economy heightens issues related to women's bodies. Marisa's disgust at her own widening body under chemo and her constant comparison to other women suggest that looking good rivals being well. Yet Marisa's antagonists are so skeletal that they look ill themselves. Hence, looking good can be looking bad. Cancer compels Marisa, who does not feel well, to exhibit what society deems attractive—looking bad, or unreasonably thin. Feeling better about herself means competing, in spite of her illness, with other women. Unsurprisingly, then, envy among women is the predominant emotion circulating around Silvano, often occurring at a table in his restaurant. Marchetto's "sour grapevine," for example, a metaphor for gossip among women, is activated "almost immediately" after Marisa begins seriously dating Silvano (50). These grapes which "are always green [with envy]" spout petty retorts about the relationship that mirror those of Marisa's rivals, such as, "It'll never last" or "All those gorgeous women he could've had—" (50). Anna Gibbs' discussion of "affect contagion" helps explain how the sour facial expressions and negative body feedback reproduce more of the same in a recipient (191). This is the "bio-neurological means by which particular affects are transmitted from body to body," explains Gibbs, using the example of the response of a smile to another's "spontaneous smile," from which I assume a frown meets another's spontaneous frown (191).[13]

The competition swirling among New York City's glamour-conscious set grooms such an ugly demeanor among such pretty (but petty) women. Marisa is keenly aware of their satisfaction if she were to suffer chemo hair and fingernail loss, develop a sallow complexion, and gain weight. (In fact, she awakens aghast one morning to find herself akin to a Mankoff cartoon, stippled with a skin irritation from one of her cancer drugs.) Marisa's battles are against both cancer and the possible ousting from the "it" community as a seemingly unsightly cancer patient. Waples notes that women with cancer are expected to adhere to a "culturally emplotted narrative of survival," like an "American entrepreneur who *achieves* survival status through toughness, optimism, and attitude" ("Avatars, Illness, and Authority" 171). *Cancer Vixen* upends this plot trajectory by exteriorizing cancer's negativity through Marisa's narcissism. If her insides are ugly and sick, at least her outside will be beautifully, attractively maintained, aligning herself away from communities of breast-cancer-afflicted women and against the grain of the "model of many other breast cancer memoirs" (Waples 171). But as Waples's self-aware narcissist (174), she maintains her position in a morally mediocre crowd. If hyperbolic negative reactions to cancer are normalized in *Cancer Vixen*, so, too, does the narrative render acceptable the many ways in which women naturalize the cultural cancer of acceptable beauty standards. Those stricken with disease or who cannot live up to these exceptionally high standards are denounced. Marisa in remission is eventually made well, but she does not act well in refusing to rise above the hurtful triviality of her social sisters.

In contrast, Ann hides nothing; she exposes what Marisa conceals—vanity—contributing to how the narratives work in tandem. Glamorous, rich, and popular, she steps on everybody and everything to work her way to the top despite her higher self's acknowledgment that this attitude keeps her, morally, at the bottom. The characters Marisa and Ann arrive at vastly different conclusions about themselves in relation to others, providing an intriguing affective comparison between the two characters' growth or stasis. Marisa's sincere explanation of her changes, that she's "not the same petty person I was before cancer . . . I'm coming from a higher place" (201), is undercut by a cartoonish buoyancy in word and image. The reader notes, however, that she remains pretty throughout her chemotherapy and other cancer treatments. Holmes calls Marchetto's tone "breezier" than other cancer narratives and "proceeds to mix cancer and couture in the snappy style and high production values of the fashion magazine" (158). In a review of several graphic pathographies in the journal *Literature and Medicine*, Hillary Chute calls *Cancer Vixen* "irritating" because of its preoccupation with women's beauty and body shape ("Review" 416) but points out that graphic protagonist Marisa knows she is shallow and narcissistic (416) and that because of this flippant perspective on a serious topic, the narrative is refreshingly unlike other cancer narratives (417). While Marchetto employs the same drawing style in *Ann Tenna*, Ann's final plunge into misery—her turning point—occurs on stark black pages. The reformed Ann who emerges from that darkness, batting her three-inch-long eyelashes dusted with sparkles, still may seem a comically ineffective role model for other women, but the gleam in her eye suggests otherwise as she "beams" goodwill around the world. The circulation of Ann's heightened self-aspiration to do good for its own sake defies Marisa's continued transactional impulse in *Cancer Vixen*, where looking fabulous always trades on those who look comparatively ugly.

Cancer Vixen and *Ann Tenna* together expose the impossible social expectations levied against women, whether ill or healthy. Marisa fears weight gain caused by some cancer drugs, for getting fat may exclude her from the "it" group, perhaps propelling Silvano toward a leaner "it" woman. Marchetto depicts Marisa's rivals as anorexically thin: Is her depiction a compliment in this competivized world of women's competitions against being overweight or an insult, as Marchetto's depicted emaciated "look" is truly unattractive? Either way, *Cancer Vixen* leaves the reader to ponder Marisa's positive estimation of women's negative self-imaging. Being thin is "in," attractive and included. Yet the coupling of caustic attitudes with skeletal women's bodies suggest how one unfortunately nurtures the other. Interestingly, the slightly chubby Silvano receives no comments about his (over)weight. In fact, the narrative insists on his captivatingly good looks despite it or perhaps even because of it. Additionally, through Marisa's naturalized hyperbolic reactions to cancer that are normalized throughout, they render acceptable the many ways in which women naturalize the cultural "cancer" or pathography of so-called beauty. Those women stricken by disease who cannot maintain society's expected beauty standards are visually denounced. Marisa's words and actions imply that the "good" approach to enduring the daily trials of cancer drugs produce negative assumptions about those who cannot make themselves look good. Ann abandons her bad attitude but is permitted a recuperation of her good looks. Had she retained permanent visual scarring, would she have climbed to the heights of SuperAnn? The two graphic narratives extol the cultural acceptance of "good" and beauty as mutually exclusive even as its figuration continues to be bad for women.

The Reboot: Imminence and Apology

While Ahmed argues emotions' circularity between and among subjects, Lauren Berlant addresses the place of "imminence" in a theory of affect she calls "cruel optimism" (97). Let us cycle Marchetto's narratives through Berlant's affective theory, in which yearning for an object of desire or state of being (rich, independent, healthy) exists "in *advance* of its loss" (emphasis in original, Berlant 94). The longing to attain what one does not have and what one assumes will improve life, love, psychic health, or corporeality exists in "imminence" (97), between what one lacks and what one wants. This "moment of suspension" (103) is "a space of potential liveness that is not a space on which anything can be built" (105). Marisa, or anybody in good health for that matter, unconsciously accepts the benefits of vigorous and pain-free existence long before becoming sick. The knowledge of having cancer marks the condition of being cancer-free a desired position. Not yet in a state of remission from cancer, hence "with" cancer, Marisa exists in a state of imminence, between being the healthy woman she (thought she) was and the healthy woman she hopes to be again. In Berlant's analysis, these "suspensions" often reveal defeat bound up in "the promises that had clustered as people's objects of desire" (97).[14]

Both graphic narratives agree that environmental toxins may be exterior causes for disease (but assuredly not causes for arrogance).[15] I return to Lorde, quoted earlier, in which she exhorts "the need for every woman to live a considered life" (57) so women can become intolerant to destructive narratives driving other- and self-assessment (57). These controls are not only clinical imperatives (a breast prosthetic to normalize a woman's body after a mastectomy) but also harmful environmental incursions. Both of Marchetto's characters muse about what they breathe, eat, and put on their skin as unconditionally important to their health and well-being. Marisa wonders if the dust from the collapsed Twin Towers in September of 2011 poisoned her, or perhaps it is New York's ubiquitous pollution. The reformed Ann imagines a line of beauty products made from organic fruits and vegetables: edible, nontoxic cosmetics.

Indeed, both Marisa and Ann are thin, beautiful, and fabulously adorned, making it difficult to judge Ann as more accepting than Marisa of others who are not on the one hand. On the other, her rectification of past wrongdoings, even if only apologizing, sets the stage for a different kind of happiness. Perhaps she can channel that to all of her "sisters" on earth, so "every woman can live a considered life" per Lorde (57), so women can become "less and less willing to tolerate those conditions unaltered [conditions or environments that cause cancer], or to passively accept external and destructive controls over our lives and our identities" (58).

In this chapter, I considered how social and medical scripts about "facing" cancer and about women's bodies are affective. Through the women protagonists of *Cancer Vixen* and *Ann Tenna*, I demonstrated how emotions circulate as affective economies to create divisions, injuries, justifications or self- and other healing. I unpacked the institutionalized systems to which Marisa conscripts herself in fighting cancer and the cultural scripts that Ann must curb in learning to live a considered life. The graphic pathographies seemingly collude over what culturally described good women do in less-than-ideal situations. They overturn expected archives of women and illness, women and beauty. They set the stage for the following chapter on women and aging. In acceding to aging as invalidating and accepting eldercare as part and parcel of women's domestic duties, out of obligation or love, we inadvertently affirm them as such: women's duties. The consequences, again for women, of subscribing to these cultural narratives are confronted in chapter 3.

Chapter 3

Aging by Frames

Thready Lines, Haptic Images, and Institutions of Care in Chast's *Can't We Talk About Something More Pleasant?* and Farmer's *Special Exits*

Unsurprisingly, graphic narratives about aging are less abundant than those about illness. Aging's inevitability for everybody can present a highly disagreeable and frightening life stage, whereas illness often strikes randomly, and we can avoid or even control some ills through adjustments to medicine, diet, and exercise.[1] This chapter looks at two graphic narratives about aging parents as illustrated by their middle-aged caregivers. Roz Chast's memoir *Can't We Talk About Something More Pleasant?* and Joyce Farmer's *Special Exits: A Graphic Memoir* depict daughters tending to elderly parents. Their tasks, they show us, are overwhelmingly challenging. For family caregivers administering to an often-uncooperative ill spouse or impaired parent, perhaps simultaneously working, looking after their own families, and navigating the complicated medical industrial complex—we expect they might be understandably cranky. Caregivers, like patients who draw manifestations of their illnesses on the page, corral positive, therapeutic energy from the artistic act of cartooning as both self-care and testimony.

This chapter charts caregivers' responses to witnessing aging, sometimes uncomfortably so. It critiques the socially accepted notion that care provided by women, here by comics avatars Roz and Laura, is "dependency work," borrowing from Eva Feder Kittay, tethered to women and passed from one generation to the next (2). Women are morally obligated to care for the elderly (and the sick, impaired) when they (the aged) eventually cannot care for themselves, she argues. "But the obligations owed" to those women who are "forced to care," the title of Evelyn Nakano Glenn's study of caregiving in America, who minister to others without requisite recognition and compensation, is a social justice issue.[2] I inquire into the following: Which subjects are cared for, how, and by whom? What and how do these graphic narratives contribute to representations of senescence? When artists draw their autobiographical encounters with the elderly, are they creating new images or cementing static ones?

Aging as a Taboo Subject

For Hiromi Goto, author of *Shadow Life* (illustrated by Ann Xu) about the fictional Kumiko Saito, an aging, bisexual, Japanese Canadian woman, compelling portrayals of aging women are scarce: "Representations of older women as interesting, heroic, powerful, and complex are not common in popular culture. Mainstream media often figure older women in clichéd roles, and ageism often frames them as the punchline of a joke" ("Author's Note," *Shadow Life*, n.p.). I will return to *Shadow Life* at the chapter's conclusion because if, for "the sighted . . . seeing is believing," states Goto in her "Author's Note," what might need *unseeing* in the visual representations about, specifically, aging women (n.p.)? As Chast's graphic narrative irritably intones, "At some point, we were all going to have to deal with this ***aging*** thing" (emphasis in original 10).

Graphic pathography more safely (or accommodatingly) addresses aging *in concert with* disease, as often depicted and narrated by family caregivers, rather than as a stand-alone topic.[3] For example, the subtitle of Sarah Leavitt's *Tangles* announces *A Story About Alzheimer's, My Mother, and Me.* Dana Walrath also tackles her mother's decline from Alzheimer's in *Aliceheimer's: Alzheimer's Through the Looking Glass.* Aneurin Wright illustrates tending to his father in home hospice, who is dying from emphysema in his *Things to Do in a Retirement Home Trailer Park . . . When You're 29 and Unemployed.*[4] These works present the troubling, challenging, painful, and eventually deadly afflictions of Alzheimer's, emphysema, and dementia, while so few others focus on a disease-free aging process. Taking up residence in a diseased state of senior citizenship remains the bad subject of good (young) life. Furthermore, because all but Wright's graphic narrative depict women tending to senescent parents, the works inquire into cultural scripts binding gender to this intimate kind of work and, as we will see, to the dissemination of family culture and lore from women to women.

Elderly but as-yet healthy parents in Roz's and Farmer's works fear the aging process, as it is freighted by circulating stigma. That anxiety appears in the repurposing of a phrase Chast's father used whenever his daughter hoped to discuss end-of-life issues. He would implore, "Can't we talk about something more pleasant?"[5] In its recycled mode as the title of Chast's comics memoir, it resounds sarcastically, signaling Roz's often astringent attitude toward aging's antics, and, eventually her parents' frightening bouts in the hospital until their deaths. Farmer's *Special Exits* is a semiautobiographical narrative about the autographic protagonist Laura's confrontation with and loving attention to the declining health of her biological father's second wife, Rachel.[6] Chast's and Farmer's memoirs adhere to two genres—comedy and realism, respectively—that participate in their own shaping of readerly attitudes toward aging and death. Chast and Farmer seem in relative agreement about how the lack of financially feasible and compassionate housing for the elderly contributes to their own perspectives, wrought by frustration about aging in America, a social justice issue. Also of significance is addressing the ethics of telling narratives about others' bodies, those embodied subjects who cannot (after death) nor may not appreciate a memoir written or drawn about them. Both Chast and Farmer, then, are entangled in depicting what G. Thomas Couser calls "vulnerable subjects," the title of one of his books, which questions whose best interests are served by representations of the disabled by the abled-bodied.[7] None of the featured parents in Chast's and Farmer's comics expresses knowledge of their appearance in a graphic narrative. Additionally, both Chast and Farmer created and published their graphic narratives after their parents' deaths. Thus, the representations are the artists' unique depiction of their parents' processes of aging and death, unmediated by their parents' input. They focus on their own authorial views and childhood memories of their elders. *Can't We Talk* and *Special Exits* depict affective afterlives of parental aging on the comics avatars of Chast and Farmer. Theirs are memoirs of a kind of artistic self-permission, leveled at nearly every memoir, I assume, in which speaking of elderly kin in relation to themselves is to speak of themselves while drawing another.[8]

Extravagance and Pragmatism: Artistic Style Unpacked

Aging is culturally overdetermined in a society that fears it and concomitantly practices ageism. Hollywood scripts around the filter-less, petulant, and childish octogenarian abound. Aging men often desperately attempt to stave off the inevitable (assumed lack of virility) or are determined to accom-

plish what life has thus far denied them (fulfill a now stereotyped bucket list). To submit gracefully to these changes might not lend themselves to a blockbuster Hollywood story, thus we spin culture's anxieties about aging into the super senior who refuses being tethered to societal assumptions to "act their age." They are asked to tone it down, rein themselves in. Youth, however, is allowed its bouts of exuberance against the expected mellowing of the senior. While these characters certainly express our culture's fears of what it means, for example, to lose one's sexual drive or to face some senescent-driven immobility, their hyperbole, especially mapped onto aging, virile men, creates a gender-driven narrative suggesting that older women face different challenges. Are these challenges caring for others or receiving care as aging adults themselves, inquire Chast's and Farmer's comics about aging parents.

Both Chast's and Farmer's graphic narratives illustratively attend to their aging parents through radically different art styles and narrative voices. In this section, I examine how Chast's and Farmer's styles and focal points contribute to tone, meaning, and focus. Who are the subjects of these autographics, I ask, the elderly or their daughters as caregivers? And if the latter over the former, then what do we, as readers, learn about aging that is new, that deviates from Hollywood scripts? Before exploring how each unique "hand" signifies, I provide their publication history as context.

Chast's narrative traffics in the humor of her signature *New Yorker* cartoons, in circulation since 1978. Her *modus operandi* are typical short vignettes with punchlines, a form exemplified in the short, interrelated comics scenarios of *Can't We Talk*. The signature emotional register in the latter is histrionic; her parents' daily habits, schedules, and limited range of self-defined acceptable foods continuously exasperate cartoon avatar Roz. She finds her aging parents personally debilitating and catastrophically monotonous, to themselves and to her. At the same time, her consistent one-panel *New Yorker* cartoons long in circulation (an artistic form or a monotonous one?) are themselves based on a routinized publishing schedule appearing with exacting regularity—forty-seven times a year. The irony and defiant attitudes prevalent in *Can't We Talk* appeared in her earlier acerbic critiques of Underground (alternative) comix's sexism in the 1960s and 1970s, influencing her tone and style. Readers not only might recognize her trademark drawing hand but also then anticipate and welcome panels saturated with predicated derision. *Can't We Talk*, for example, could be read as a wink and nod to those middle-agers like Roz who find themselves nurturing aging, seemingly eccentric parents at whom one must laugh to keep from crying in despair. Overall, I conjecture that through the graphic narrative's few but rare tender images, Chast is not against aging—she is no ageist—but rather is opposed to how her parents have aged and is angered by a society where health care and assisted living are financially prohibitive for so many.

On the one hand, Chast's distinctive thready hand[9] captures the fragility of her aging parents whose vociferous refusals of assistance appear in speech balloons made "loud" by underlined and bolded words, by oversized characters, and through plenty of exclamation points.[10] On the other, because scenarios are replete with sweat drops, motion lines, squiggles, and other indicators of Roz's unceasing exasperation in the face of her relentlessly resistant parents, *Can't We Talk* depicts seniors who are tougher than the seeming fragility depicted by Chast's scratchy, hand-drawn lines. Rather, character heft, font sizes, bolding and underlining, and other artistic elements express Chast's views of her parents. Elizabeth, her mother, is intense, formidable; her verbal opinions and commands often burst from the confines of speech balloons or panel frames, accompanied by copious exclamation points. She can blow you away! Readers easily detect the weight of her "big" emotions without the aid of words. When agitated, Elizabeth's cartoon figure enlarges, panel by panel on the page. Her perpetually open mouth, yelling more often than talking, channels her wired personality. Her father, George, who is depicted as the meeker of the married couple and eventually develops "senile dementia" (28), is constantly on edge around his wife. In one of Chast's visual comparisons between them, Elizabeth "was built like a fire hydrant" (55). George stands as a diminished figure to her right, trembling in her shadow: "Indeed you are!" he mumbles (55) (fig. 4).

The scratchy, frenetic quality of Chast's line channels less a sense of aging's frailty than a constant irritation, as when Roz becomes increasingly agitated, whether desperately seeking a convenient parking space near her mother's hospital in New York City (141) or sending invisible anger waves at a nurse's back (63). Chast's comment early in the graphic memoir, "I wasn't great as a caretaker, and they [my parents] weren't great at being taken care of," notes that already existing family dispositions would be exacerbated by Roz's penchant for hyperbole, amplifying her parents' mounting inabilities and their consistent intransigence to all suggestions meant to ameliorate

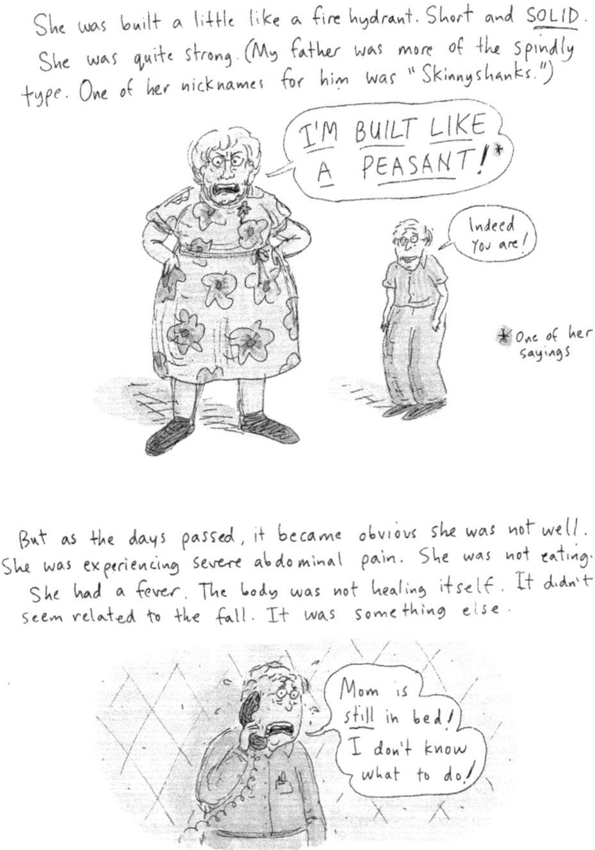
She was built a little like a fire hydrant. Short and SOLID. She was quite strong. (My father was more of the spindly type. One of her nicknames for him was "Skinnyshanks.")
I'M BUILT LIKE A PEASANT!*
Indeed You are!
* One of her sayings
But as the days passed, it became obvious she was not well. She was experiencing severe abdominal pain. She was not eating. She had a fever. The body was not healing itself. It didn't seem related to the fall. It was something else.
Mom is still in bed! I don't know what to do!

Fig. 4 | Elizabeth is formidable and loud, overshadowing her husband, George. From Roz Chast, *Can't We Talk About Something More Pleasant?*, p. 55. Copyright © Roz Chast 2014, Bloomsbury Publishing Inc. / Used by permission of The Wiley Agency LLC.

escalating challenges (16). Thus is Chast's graphic narrative an emphatically noisy one. No tepid reaction exists. One is either anxiously awaiting an explosion or living through it. Panels overwrought with mood and tone are the graphic narrative's soundtrack. Her style exhibits a good cartoonist's uncanny ability to find humor not only in the mundane (wherein molehills grow into farcical mountains) but also in the monumental (having children, becoming gravely ill, facing death).

At first, we might assume Roz is the butt of her own punchlines, wherein she tolerates the tedium of her elderly parents' obstinacy and insufferable routinization. But her humor also is drollery directed at her parents, at whom we laugh for just the represented tedium of caring that Chast illustrates.

Couser reminds us that "when memoir aims at humor, readers are inclined to tolerate, even welcome, what Mark Twain called 'stretchers'" (*Memoir: An Introduction* 82). In another light, Chast's mocking tone accompanying her stretching impulse may make light of heavy end-of-life decisions. It might assist her in conceding to caring for an overbearing and loveless mother. Did she love me? Chast inquires implicitly near the narrative's conclusion (201–2). In her depictions of George, her father, drawn as perpetually under Elizabeth's thumb, Chast seems to appreciate his calm and reserved personality. Finally, that Roz has children, is married, and works as a well-respected artist on publications whose deadlines are never paused in deference to human issues like elder care, all magnify the enormous responsibilities she juggles simultaneously. Additionally, rude and inattentive hospital staff palpably impact Roz and, we assume, her husband and children, waiting in the wings while she tends to her mother and father.[11]

Farmer is known for sexually graphic work featured in *Wimmen's Comix*. Published between 1972 and 1992, it is the first comics collection addressing feminist issues, including women, sex, and sexuality. It provided the foundation from which many *Wimmen's Comix* contributors were propelled into their artistic careers. Even before its advent, however, Joyce Farmer and Lyn Chevely produced the sexually explicit *Tits and Clits* (1972–1987), considered audacious even in the counterculture of the 1970s. It enjoyed a fifteen-year run.[12] Their jointly produced *Abortion Eve* appeared shortly after the passage of *Roe v. Wade* in 1973 and is currently available in its entirety online.[13] Farmer's depiction of attentive geriatric care in *Special Exits* thus veers broadly from her other initial and "unique [even contested among women at the time] form of feminist activism" (Chadwick Roberts 1). At the same time, however, elder care and sexual well-being exist on a continuum of women's overall health. As a cartoonist, Farmer's political motivations to attend to women's welfare remain the same, only her narrative tone changes from bellicose, in her earlier work, to tender in *Special Exits*.

Unlike Chast's preference for free-form comics, Farmer adheres to a consistent eight-panel grid, two panels across, four panels down. The graphic form organizes protagonist Laura's emotionally messy care work. Her hand is a fine and detailed line. It expresses the tedium involved in caring for somebody's bodily health and hygiene on a daily basis and the ongoing chore (sometimes a labor of love and other times just sheer labor) of literally cleaning up (often people) and later cleaning out spaces of crammed "collections," a euphemism for her stepmother Rachel and biological father Lars's hoarding. Additionally, Farmer's realistic black-and-white drawings convey emotional drag, delineating clearly how the burdens of caring and cleaning wear on her. This is accomplished less through a noisy soundscape like that used by Chast, seemingly shouting at her readers, than through smell and touch. Farmer's haptic images, such as highly textured fabrics or the materiality of a household of acquired stuff, invites a kind of visual sensory experience. According to Hillary Chute, the hand-drawn form is a "sensual practice" (*Disaster Drawn* 4).[14] Additionally, Laura remarks, "Their house stinks . . . [and] cat hair is everywhere" (75), but she also lovingly sponge bathes Rachel on the couch, brushes her hair, enjoys the softness of clean flannel pajamas on her stepmother.

Farmer's scruffy, cross-hatched style effectively captures her parents' overgrown, dilapidated house, seemingly disappearing under a carpet of moss and other dusty, fuzzy plant growth that makes it stand out shabbily from the neatly kempt neighbors' lawns in their South Los Angeles location (7). When Ching, their Siamese cat, scratches clouds of fur into the air (32), the allergic Laura develops a clearly delineated rash whose bumps on her arm rival the details of Lars's five o'clock shadow (32); the dust covering Rachel's doll collection and the flowery designs on Rachel's dresses clash with the couch's equally efflorescent pattern (20). These disharmonious details demonstrate that no visual tranquility exists in *Special Exits*. Readers leave the graphic narrative with an overstimulated eye. Yet appreciating all of Farmer's detail-intensive hand endorses the enormity of Laura's caregiving labor.

If Chast's derision rehearses a disciplined emotional distance from her parents,[15] predominant mid-range, head-and-shoulder shots—no intimacy here—keep readers at a remove from Elizabeth and George's emotional interiority. One typically humorous narrative, however, allows a possible financial past history for Elizabeth's present behavior. Elizabeth's burgeoning economic mindset developed during the Depression, a memory about the scarcity of money from her frugal childhood that she cannot shake to the present day. Much to Roz's incredulity, Elizabeth buys stockings in the colors of avocado and lobster bisque—to what in her mother's wardrobe can they be paired, she intones—only because they are 80 percent reduced from the retail price, a near give-away (47). She will dye them, remarks Elizabeth, or make them into a vest for George. Roz tries to convince us that Elizabeth's outrageous parsimoniousness arises from an aspect of her personality, not from a rational response to life's challenges, such as the Depression, in which necessity trumps fashion. Thriftiness, then, passes from Elizabeth's parents to the next generation. Depicting in material form what Roz only conjures imaginatively is Chast's creative punchline: two pieces of fabric shaped like feet are stitched down each shoulder of a patchwork vest for George (47). The image, however, says more about Roz, the impatient daughter, than Elizabeth, the parsimonious mother. Her mother's common sense overall seems more acceptable than her daughter's preposterous amplification of the situation. Might Elizabeth be equally rankled by her insensitive (irrational?) daughter? As if an appreciative nod to these dynamics, in the vignette's concluding panel Roz draws herself trailing her mother, who is moving from the center of the panel to the right, a Western-centric direction suggesting forward motion, leaving Roz behind. Elizabeth gets the last gesture and the last word. Toting multiple packages of vastly reduced lobster bisque–colored stockings in hand, she quips, "Waste not, want not" (47).

Farmer addresses similar issues, such as her elders' obstinacy, incontinence, and memory loss, but with gentle common sense and evenhanded patience. *Special Exits* is divided into fourteen chapters that chart Rachel's slow decline from moderate healthiness to death. Even if Rachel is not Laura's biological mother, the latter is compelled out of love for her father, who loves Rachel, to care for her stepmother as she incrementally becomes immobile and finally impaired, confined to the couch. Chast depicts Roz as the younger, always more able subject against that of her always-already aged parents. Farmer, however, uses the arthrological connection of mirroring across panels to democratize the experiences of the young and the old. The former humorizes; the latter humanizes. Thierry Groensteen describes arthrology as the process by which icons and images systemically create meaning across panels and pages (*System of Comics* 21–23). For example, in chapter 3 of *Special Exits*, Laura, Rachel, and Lars all fall at some point in the duration of the diegesis, but under disparate circumstances and to different reactions: Laura, first, while dancing with her partner; Rachel in the midst of what looks like fainting; and Lars while chasing Ching, the cat, in the backyard. The characters are visually unified and equalized across their various prone positions. Caught unexpectedly by gravity, each understands that particular feeling of being upended. The surprise of sudden inversion lends a generous, discretionary response to considerations of being clumsy (Laura) or frail (Lars and Rachel). *Special Exits*'s Laura, Lars, and Rachel, of vastly divergent ages, genders, and bodily abilities, experience similar situations by which Farmer fashions an equal plane of humanity among them. In contrast, *Can't We Talk* traffics in hierarchy from the first page, pitting Roz's parents as increasingly irrational against their daughter's self-proclaimed lucidity.

In *Can't We Talk*, who makes claims on where our sympathy falls when "managing" elder care? Does it lie with Roz or with Elizabeth and George?

Is Roz pinpointing challenges in elder care or laughing at the elders in that care? The vignettes, I argue, eventually solicit sympathy for the generally harried and judgmental Roz when coupled with depictions of the mounting difficulties of care that are embedded in labyrinthine insurance policies and perplexing health care system protocols, to be undertaken later in this chapter's conclusion on women and care giving. They confuse even a younger generation armed with financial expertise in the growing confuse-opoly of the health *care* industry. Readers are encouraged to rail against the system, not against Elizabeth and George. We are on Roz's side because we, too, might one day be overwhelmed by the Kafkaesque medical industrial complex.

Amid the frenzy of care that renders *Can't We Talk* a collection of energized images, however, the graphic narrative contains an emotionally raw and telling scene that necessitates discussion. Its tenderness tamps the graphic narrative's intensity, provides some rationale for Roz's affectional hardness, and reveals heretofore unfulfilled longing. In this 228-page graphic narrative, we learn only by page 201 that Elizabeth never hoped to be closer to Roz, as Roz hoped to become to Elizabeth. And near Elizabeth's death, Roz asks during a visit, "Do you want me to stay or should I go?" "It doesn't matter," replies Elizabeth. "I left her room," writes Roz, "walked to my car. When I got in, I cried. The bellowing quality of the sobbing and the depth of the sadness I felt surprised me. I was angry, too. Why hadn't she tried harder to know me? But I knew: if there had ever been a time in my relationship with my mother for us to get to know one another—and that's a very big 'if'—that time had long since passed" (202).

However, near the graphic narrative's conclusion, Chast suffuses drawings of her mother, moments after her death, with a gentleness not depicted earlier. Against a background of muted yellow, Elizabeth's peaceful face and still form unsettle the former frenzied energy and bold colors of the graphic pathography (211–22). If Elizabeth's mouth was once an orifice for shouting, arguing, or complaining, in these sketches it becomes the aperture between life and death—taking in air and expelling it, until the life-sustaining rhythm stops. She is so lovingly illustrated that her face and mouth capture the reader's full attention. Chast's delicate, crosshatched strokes outline the soft curves of her mother's slight body beneath the hospital coverings, evoking sensation and tender sensibility at once.

Chast employs what Davide Panagia calls "visual tactility," which he defines as "collapsing the experience of seeing and that of touching" (109). He states, "The emphasis on the face as a site of such representational potency [between the realms of life and death] is also significant because it imposes on the viewer a kind of physical and psychological nudity, the idea that at the moment when life encounters death, all our resources are at once exhausted and displayed on the surface" (103). Chast's drawing hand here "touches" her mother's fragility and the reader. Touch is defined as emotion as well as a drawing style that differs significantly from the harsher "hand" abundantly used throughout *Can't We Talk*. In this delicate depiction of her mother's waning life and moment of death, Chast allows viewers to "feel" much less the weight of Chast's predominantly angry narrative throughout than the levity of her relief. Readers move with the narrative diegesis and are moved by the force of Chast's poignant images, affected by what Panagia calls an "aesthetic experience" (109).

In the epilogue, Chast returns to full-color images with a sting, restoring a derisive Roz as she giddily places her parents (or their sacks of cremains) in the closet: the phrase "I like having my parents in my closet" (227) is mitigated by "Every time I open its door . . . I think of them" (227). Yet the former, disquieting images of her dying mother remain with the reader, subtly enigmatic, asking readers to confront finitude: "What occurs after death? Where do the deceased go? Reason as definitive thinking, especially in Roz's views throughout, is replaced by the inconclusive. What better way to destabilize medical and political absolutism than through questioning the existence of a realm beyond reach, beyond human definition and categorization? What better conclusion to a graphic pathography pitting the rational, the practical, and the senseless, as attributed to Elizabeth and George, by the seemingly level-headed Roz herself?

Drawing Out Atmosphere Among a Life's Collection of Stuff

In *Comics and the Body: Drawing, Reading, and Vulnerability*, Eszter Szép addresses not only how the mark-making artist uses her hand, an embodied reaction to depicted vulnerability, but also how the reading body performs "kinaesthetic empathy" (a term she borrows from Laura Marks 137). Szép argues for the "performative and embodied nature" of reading comics (139), which she calls "feeling the line" (141), a haptic affinity with my own readings on the relationship between materiality and environment in *Special Exits* and *Can't We Talk*.

If, for Chast, "the key sensual experience is seeing rather than touching or holding . . . objects" (Jenkins n.p.), Farmer's detailed drawings in *Special Exits* depict objects' materiality, offering the narrative a haptic, sensory quality; they exhibit an expressive range across her works, explicitly through the visual representation of the senses. Farmer adores texture, from ribbed turtlenecks to striped flannel pajamas, from fringed silk scarves to brittle, drying hair. Her *modus operandi* is an invocation of the senses through the material. Farmer's black-and-white drawings that use more realism than Chast's caricatures convey Laura's concern for her aging parents less through sound (less through Chast's "noisy" and frenetic panels) than through smell and touch. Illustrated texture relates to loving care. Farmer's detailed ink drawings permit us to "see" how a checked flannel nightgown, after a warm sponge bath, might feel soft and comforting against Rachel's sensitive skin. Farmer's attention to Laura's sense of touch, here, signals tender feelings toward her father and stepmother.

The flowery living room couch and matching chair, whose Jacquard weave upholstery is animated by Farmer's detailed ink work, sits at the heart of Rachel and Lars's house. Farmer returns repeatedly to this couch, homing in on its raised petunia pattern as it eventually becomes the most convenient, central location in the house for Rachel, in her own patterned dresses, to eat, sleep, and be bathed. As Rachel diminishes in weight and mental capacity, the couch gains the accoutrements of care: Laura covers the cushions, readies blankets nearby (including a stack for Rachel's sitting comfort), perches a stuffed bear on the backing, and provides magazines at arm's length. Loving acts of bodily care and conversation occur on this piece of furniture, from sitting with Rachel to chat, to filing and painting her fingernails, to gently brushing her hair. The panels thus cluttered with clashing patterns, fabrics, textures, and household things propose intimacy, not disarray or discord, while crowded panels in other graphic narratives often indicate chaos, as in the *horror vacui* of Julie Doucet's *My New York Diary*; or the compression of a Holocaust survivor's history and a son's artistic grappling with it in Art Spiegelman's *Maus*; or in the quivering life of the forest mirroring a vicious virus spreading rapidly among sexually active youth in Charles Burns's *Black Hole*.[16] In Katie Mullins's discussion of aging as experienced by character Lou in Jeff Lemire's graphic narrative trilogy *Essex County*, she argues that "it is Lou's body—his sensory perception, physical experience, and gestures—that helps him to remember his past and tell his story but which also enables him to connect to the external world" (33). Mullins argues that Lou's memory returns him cognitively to past locations and contributes to his sense of agency in his aging body. Panel density and arrangement in Farmer's *Special Exits*, as well as highly textured images created through endless strokes of the pen, all contribute to fabricating atmosphere, perhaps stifling on the one hand, but suffused with loving emotion on the other that constantly returns us to Rachel's aging body. Farmer's hand offers Rachel subjectivity and agency.

Farmer strategically illustrates tactile images to demonstrate how her family teaches each other, a form of influence markedly different than Chast's often negatively affective emotions circulating from parents to daughter and back. When Ching first enjoys a belly rub from Laura before unexpectedly biting her hand, Lars instructs Laura how to approach Ching better next time. He establishes rules of engagement between Laura and Ching to suggest similar guidelines necessary between Laura and her parents. In the vignette's final panel, Lars shows the Band-Aids on his arms that conceal former Ching-induced wounds, demonstrating that he, too, is not always prudent enough with the temperamental cat that now dozes peacefully on his lap. These seventeen panels of *Special Exits*'s initial vignette focus on the three characters' emotional and tactile relationship with Ching in order to inaugurate Farmer's graphic pathography about loving and accidentally wounding by turns.

A common reference point in texts about the elderly who are tended to by their children is the cluttered family house in which fifty or more years of living results in an accumulation of stuff. These collections, a positively inflected term, often are deemed the results of what less charitable descendants negatively regard as hoarding, especially if they are charged with tediously sorting through them. In his study of the toll these possessions might take on adult children strapped with culling them, Henry Jenkins calls the gleaning process a "divestment ritual" (n.p.). The paraphernalia occupying the house invites articulations about how things, and subsequently how a lived life, come to matter. In Chast's chapter 10, "The Old Apartment," Roz makes aesthetic use of found objects that have survived, even seemingly multiplied, over forty-eight years in the family home. In an unusual artistic move, Roz provides a photo gallery, in the center of the text, of some of her parents' vintage objects that provide glimpses into their younger selves. But it is not the items themselves that inspire close consideration but rather Roz's thoughtful arrangements of them: neatly aligning a collection of her mother's cat-eye glasses on a page that also spotlights a vintage stapler and three electric shavers (109–18).[17] Andrew Kunka claims that the photos provide concrete evidence of the "obsolete stuff" Roz finds amid the "sheer level of clutter" in her parents' home (72, 73).[18] Referring to it as "clutter" or dismissing it as "obsolete stuff" repudiates the sentimental value the items hold.[19] In fact, these lovingly arranged and photographed objects are a rare instance in the entire graphic narrative of fond reminiscence, notwithstanding Chast's images of her mother moments after death discussed above. Against Kunka's assessment, I argue that having already established her parents' peculiarity, the photos are less about representing Elizabeth and George's quirkiness than about Roz's surprising nostalgia in a graphic narrative leaning toward resentment and irritation. In addition, the flat quality of the photographs against the splintery artistic hand of Chast's drawings is a jarring juxtaposition. The photographs take us out of the loud, hand-drawn diegesis for a few pages, like a breath of air, before plunging us back into the literal and figurative fray of her noisy drawings. Perhaps the stuff of "the old apartment" that contributes to its claustrophobia is also inadvertently calming. The paraphernalia of Farmer's cramped panels include the aforementioned stacked blankets, and also boxes, oil lamps, magazines, dolls, and other accumulated and accumulating fragments, many of which are storied, of Lars and Rachel's collective lives (fig. 5).

Clutter might be dusty junk for some, but for Laura and her parents, it contains inherited family stories, the afterlives of material objects that bring the family together in remembrance. Farmer relates anecdotes of three specific items, Rachel's agate-and-gold necklace (passed down from her deceased father) (91), an 1845 pistol that once belonged to his Danish immigrant grandpa (94–95), and a Civil War–era rifle used in the Spanish-American War by his Uncle Paul (99). The proliferation of stuff in the panel frames routes readers away from endowing them with negative connotations of clutter and toward augmenting their value as family narratives. Material objects reflect an intimacy shared among Laura, Rachel, and Lars. Laura organizes them to create a cleaner, healthier space for her parents. Roz, on the other hand, in carefully arraying formerly haphazard collections after her parents' deaths, seeks order from chaos. She regulates that which she can—material objects left behind—while her parents' perceived erratic behavior falls well beyond her organizational ken.

Not Against Aging but Opposing Its Institutions

In *The Body at Risk: Photography of Disorder, Illness, and Healing*, Carol Squiers cites a study estimating that by 2030 the population of the United States aged sixty-five and older will outnumber those under twenty (193). The aging of America is a cause of great concern for its youth: Who will care for seniors? Who will oversee the ethical and compassionate management of their living spaces when family can no longer assist them at home? At this concluding juncture, assessing whose view, between Roz's and Laura's, is more merciful

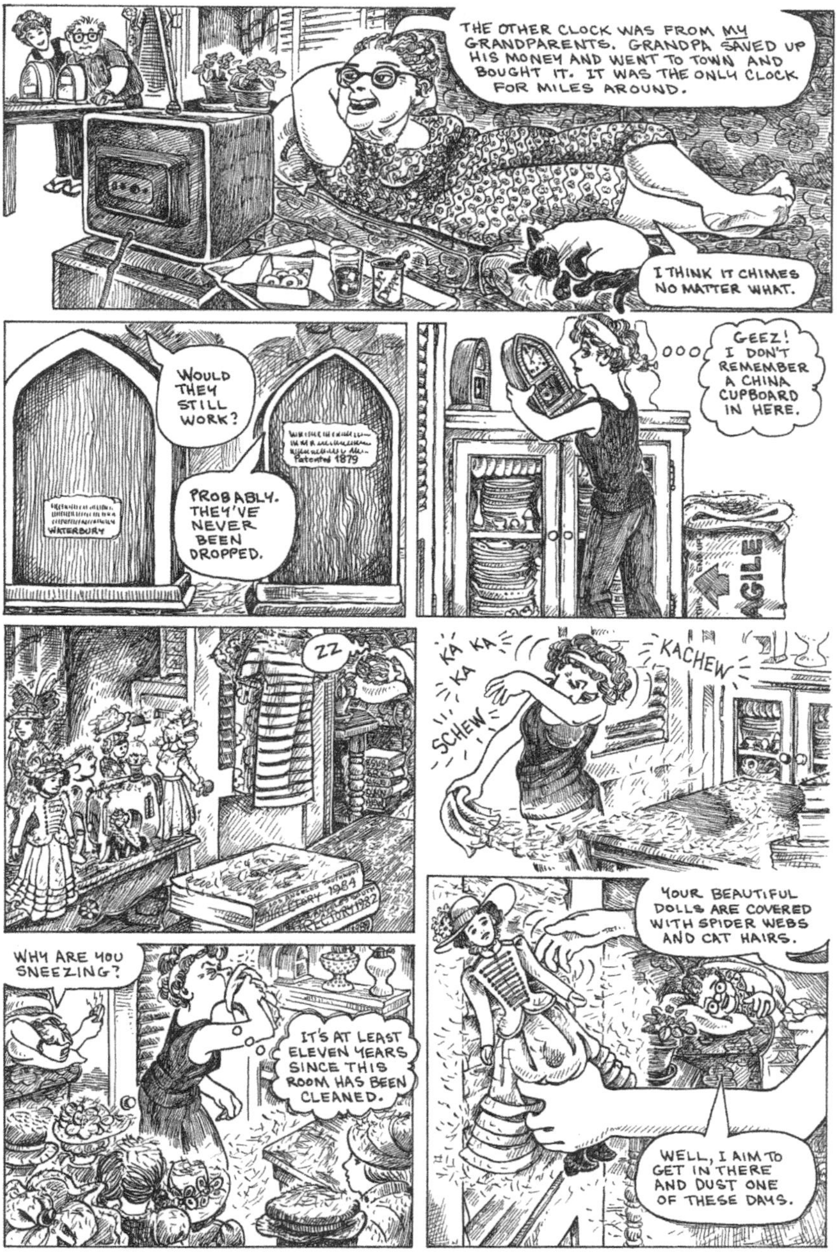
THE OTHER CLOCK WAS FROM MY GRANDPARENTS. GRANDPA SAVED UP HIS MONEY AND WENT TO TOWN AND BOUGHT IT. IT WAS THE ONLY CLOCK FOR MILES AROUND.
I THINK IT CHIMES NO MATTER WHAT.
WOULD THEY STILL WORK?
PROBABLY. THEY'VE NEVER BEEN DROPPED.
WATERBURY
Patented 1879
OOO
GEEZ! I DON'T REMEMBER A CHINA CUPBOARD IN HERE.
ZZ
KA KA KA
SCHEW
KACHEW
WHY ARE YOU SNEEZING?
IT'S AT LEAST ELEVEN YEARS SINCE THIS ROOM HAS BEEN CLEANED.
YOUR BEAUTIFUL DOLLS ARE COVERED WITH SPIDER WEBS AND CAT HAIRS.
WELL, I AIM TO GET IN THERE AND DUST ONE OF THESE DAYS.

Fig. 5 | Farmer's cramped panels filled with textured paraphernalia, p. 20. Copyright © Joyce Farmer. Courtesy of Fantagraphics Books (www.fantagraphics.com).

or sympathetic as my readings may have suggested, is less important than attending to the consequences of a national "care crisis" (Glenn 183). Roz, noting the indignities her mother suffers in the hospital as she awaits death, finds them "beyond imagining" (163). No wonder caring for them at home seems more appealing for her despite the toll it takes. Near the conclusion to *Special Exits*, Laura and Lars cope with one escalating stress around Rachel after another. Laura quips that Rachel's "needs are killing him [Lars], but he [Lars] won't let me hire help" (135). Lars maintains what Evelyn Nakano Glenn calls an age-old ideology that "in-home caring labor" remains a familial obligation, concretized in the "private family realm" (149). In her *Forced to Care*, this private family matter remains separate from the public "market" because of deep-seated cultural norms, encouraged by men like Lars, that such care is an altruistic, unremunerable resource, usually provided by women (149).[20] Despite over a century of legal battles attempting to overturn generally unpaid or grossly underpaid home care, Glenn claims that such home-care roles are reinforced and sustained by interrelated factors, many reliant on gender expectations: historical precedents; economically convenient reliance on unpaid women's labor; ideological assumptions about women's work as wives, partners, and mothers; continued unequal pay between men and women in the workforce; a sense of duty; a lack of other financial options; and love (6). Thus, Lars refuses to hire help because of precedent—women are best suited and thus expected to perform this care—or perhaps because of Laura's unvoiced but enacted filial piety, and because of the benefits to his pocketbook: Laura's labor is unremunerated. Attentive to Rachel's needs and his own, in that order, he might not deign to acknowledge the physical and psychological toll that care giving takes on his daughter and how it cobbles her participation to earn a salary in the public market, impoverishing her own pocketbook.

Affordable quality eldercare options are social justice issues "as recognized and valued," claims Glenn (188–90). In an episode featuring an angry Laura, she tells the hospital director that her [now] blind stepmother fell out of bed and broke her hip because an employee "left her bed rail down," and "your facility is responsible for her situation" (146). While in former pages Farmer never includes the thought balloons of characters other than herself, in this vignette she allows the hospital director an unvoiced "I hate this" to emanate from his head (146). Both Farmer and Chast illustrate the compounding pressures of finding a "good" senior residence, wading through insurance paperwork, and advocating tirelessly for parents who cannot do so themselves. In a telling scene, Laura tells her husband Art, "The folks are having a hard time taking care of themselves. They're both afraid of 'homes.'" He replies, "You can't blame them" (34). If we are unable to find a solution to a dearth of excellent, respectful care providers against a rise of those necessitating such ministration, Glenn argues, (women) family and friends will be "overburdened" with care duties, "sacrificing their own health and well-being" (183). Attending to the aging in America must be regarded as a systemic, community challenge, not a singular (or familial) individual one.[21]

In the fictional work *Shadow Life* by author Goto and artist Xu, we see aging Japanese Canadian protagonist Kumiko Saito fending off encroaching death, depicted as a voracious black spider and a watery, shoeless ghost that pursue her. Her children are enraged at "mami's" independence, as she chooses to stay in her apartment rather than relocating to an expensive, long-awaited room in a "nice" assisted living facility. Kumiko's imaginative solutions to staving off death are more humorous and effective at forestalling it than is bending to her children's will. She sucks death's shadow into her vacuum cleaner. "I guess I look old. I don't 'feel old' inside. Do people who see me think, 'She's an old woman?'" Kumiko asks herself (30). Goto delves into octogenarian Kumiko's thoughts, a contrasting perspective to Chast's and Farmer's positions as mere onlookers to aging (30). In the "Author's Note" in *Shadow Life*, Goto, whose past prose work *Chorus of Mushrooms* addresses women, culture, and belonging, writes, "I've seen many films about grumpy old white men, but far fewer of old women. And no mainstream North American films that center on BIPOC queer elders. I bring up film because this is the most visual form of representation that hits the eyes and minds of broad cultural demographics. For the sighted, in many ways, seeing is believing" (n.p.). *Shadow Life* un-sees those typical representations to fill Goto and the reader "with strength and direction" (n.p.).[22]

Chast and Farmer's graphic narratives obliquely reference other pending challenges, especially concerning a history of race and caregiving, race and health, mother-daughter relationships, and the future of mothering. In the collection *Revolutionary Mothering*, Alexis Pauline Gumbs asks, where is the "Black feminist position" in mother-daughter representations (21)? Gumbs's work hearkens back to not only sterilization movements across the globe looking to reduce the reproduction of black and brown babies but also to the 2005 "neo-eugenicist" words of William Bennett, former Secretary of Education, that "aborting every black baby would decrease crime" (Gumbs 20). That Black women continue to mother, both their children and their own aging mothers, begs for graphic pathography to take up these issues to fight the disparagement created in the link between "mother" and

"Black" (21) and to both critique and undo a history of the "racialization of care" (Glenn 6). Where are representations in graphic medicine by black and brown women caregivers who tend, very often, to white bodies? Who are "forced to care"? What form does care take in such an arrangement? What does creating oneself look like, as a Black woman in the realm of "motherHOOD" (a position), or that of "motherING" (sustaining work from slavery to the present moment) (emphasis in original 22)? What might these caregivers depict in concert with or against presentations by Chaz and Farmer? The pronounced absence of viewpoints by raced subjects in a medium now crowded with white women as caregiving subjects advances white women as heroic, sacrificial, overly generous at the expense of images of black and brown women who disproportionately continue to care for white bodies—at low pay, punishing weekly hours, and often without labor protections. The latter then persist as glorified helpmates in the American imaginary, but not as agential subjects in their own right. The following chapter takes the literal built spaces of the clinic as ideological arenas that care, predominantly, for white bodies.

Chapter 4

Hospital Waiting Rooms as Medicine's Sedimented Spaces

Ware's *Jimmy Corrigan* and Potts's *Good Eggs*

Graphic pathography engages in both abstract and concrete definitions of the term institution. The institution of medicine, for example, constitutes a culture and ideology that subjects of graphic pathography sometimes find, ironically, inimical to their health and well-being. The former chapter, for example, advocates for innovative eldercare institutions (as physical locations and as ideological entities), relieving children of some portion of the cultural expectation to nurture incapacitated elderly parents, often alone, through the latter's challenges of seniority, infirmity, disease, or impairment. Exhausted by other familial duties, the daughters discussed in Chast's and Farmer's work yearn for affordable and excellent care unburdened by the kinds of insensitive staff that render home care provided by family members a qualitatively better solution for elderly parents in a dearth of high-caliber outpatient facilities—yet a situation perhaps less than ideal for these busy daughters.

Graphic pathographies respond to the cultural disciplining of health, illness, and disability within specific arenas. They draw out and upon socially and culturally defined physical spaces such as sick rooms, hospital wards, wings, waiting rooms, emergency rooms (ERs).[1] Roxanne Mountford usefully suggests that space "carries with it the sediment of cultural tradition, of the social imaginary" (quoted in Dolmage 63). An institution, then, is a geographical-social dynamic. Designated medical spaces are physical locations whose staff convey knowledge and exercise medical procedures as needed; their actions and ideologies are crosshatched with cultural-social networks and conduits. The structures of medical institutions, their hierarchies and cultural practices, all frame behavior within and are influenced from (patients) without. Their mingling on the comics page visualizes layers of meanings that interact with and against each other.[2]

Waiting rooms are not only ubiquitous spaces in clinics and hospitals but, contrary to their quiet ambiance, are charged with patients' internal anxious thoughts and fretful anticipations: What will the doctor discover? How will surgery proceed? Will I be cancer-free in a year, or will I die? These anxieties as palpable energy circulate among and affect patients, their visitors, the hospital staff, inviting a closer look at these meaningful spaces that, heretofore, have received no scholarly attention. In this chapter, I put theories of space in conversation with comics' depictions of arenas in hospitals and clinics designated for waiting. Spatial and temporary flows, including obstructions to fluidity, pulse through these comics spaces. I construct an understanding of the unintentionally competitive environment of, for example, an infertility clinic's reception lounge in Phoebe Potts's *Good Eggs: A Memoir* in which some patients' inability to reproduce exacerbates an anxiety about the necessity to fulfill social expectations of providing progeny, the reproductive futurism argued by Lee Edelman. The visually cramped environment of an ER anteroom in Chris Ware's *Jimmy Corrigan: The Smartest Kid on Earth* illuminates confrontations over race and sibling responsibilities for a dying father. Comics' imagined spaces and the spaces of imagination converge among the energies of medical culture and the waiting individual, sometimes a patient, sometimes a visitor.

Numerous comics scholars argue that the medium is especially suited for representational feats that prose cannot perform.[3] Prose text requires us to move from word to word in chronological order to assemble meaning and construct the diegesis. In comics' compositional iconostasis, however, according to Andre Molotiu, "the perception of the layout of a comics page as a unified composition . . . [invites readers] to take it in at a glance" (n.p.). The possibility of a page's global view of image/s defies the necessary chronology of prose. Graphic pathographies' empaneled networks of emotion in their depictions of waiting rooms benefit from such an affordance. Comics approach to the simultaneity of time—through diachrony, synchrony, and iconostasis—is valuable here. In Thierry Groensteen's *The System of Comics*, panels create networks of meaning across a-chronological pages and comics space rather than through linear sequentialism. His spatio-topical system privileges the work of reticulation that connects icons and panels accumulatively beyond continuous, uninterrupted, serialization. In addition, Scott McCloud's chapter "Time Frames," in his *Understanding Comics*, is an illustrated introduction to how comics depict both discretely and concurrently (94–117). For McCloud, we can read a series of events that are illustrated from left to right, as if moment by moment, while also understanding that the individually depicted events might be occurring at the same time. From sexual violence to war, from genocide to addiction, comics' representational potential to record and visually report arises from its particular capacity to express time and manipulate space in service to the monumental and the habitual, the extraordinary and the traumatic . . . and the interminable hospital wait.

Waiting as a Space

Waiting rooms in life and as depicted in the featured graphic narratives of this chapter encompass and express dispositional frequencies that resonate with graphic pathography's waiting subjects. To wait is to conform to expectation. Sara Ahmed claims that we orient ourselves toward objects that allow us to perform tasks that need doing (*Queer Phenomenology* 33). Throughout her study, she uses the example of the writing table, toward which an author or illustrator turns to do her work. She orients her body toward the table at the same time that the table affords that alignment or is designed for such acclimation, exemplified by ergonomic design that assists in anatomical health vis-à-vis other necessary work tools, such as chairs and laptops. Ahmed's theories help position the waiting room as an object that transforms "time into form" (Ahmed 40). Because there exists no one-to-one correspondence between number of patients and medical providers, not everybody can be seen at the same time; waiting is an anticipated, expected ritual in medical care.[4] In a waiting room, we halt our usual activities to attend to an annual appointment, a routine check-up, a diagnosis, a prognosis, or news about a loved one. The waiting interval can be blissfully short or agonizingly long. Ahmed argues, "You bring your past encounters with you when you arrive [at an object like a writing table]" (*Queer Phenomenology* 40). A person with a former negative medical experience will apprehensively enter the waiting room affected by that prior exchange. Those with only positive experiences and diagnoses may feel less burdened by fear but also experience trepidation because medicine looks for signs of disease at the same time that it tests for health. "The fear of an illness," states Rita Charon of a patient waiting for a biopsy report, can be as uncomfortable as the illness itself (*Narrative Medicine* 44).

For Charon, a patient "inhabits a timeless enduring," which she explains as "living within and outside of time, between diachrony and synchrony" (*Narrative Medicine* 44).[5] Hence the "skirmish about waiting room time might be taken seriously," she continues, suggesting that the perpetually late physician who overlooks the anxiety of the waiting patient sends a "pervasive and powerful message" to the patient about her worth (44). The patient understands that she might linger in a chair for some time, Ahmed's anticipated "future that might or 'perhaps' will happen" (40). An arrival into waiting is freighted with a past and a future as it is also ironically an abeyance, Charon's timeless enduring. Sharing—"sharing" itself as an invisible, circulated feeling—occurs in this waiting room's analepsis and prolepsis with others whose arrivals, departures, and futures render the space a layered habitus, if only for an hour. The waiting room itself does not "have" culture; it is created in concert with subjects riven by opinions, histories, and emotions that crisscross its space. Given that waiting rooms are often a patient's introduction to clinical care, their prominent absence from prose is surprising, their occasional inclusion in comics invaluable.

Theorizing Waiting Rooms: Socio-Spatial and Socio-Topical Systems

Before comics scholarship developed its own comics-specific terminology, it often borrowed approaches from film theory, especially to address the fluidity and variability of passing time in comics' flat, static panels. It has expanded to reference semiotics, visual rhetoric, and cultural criticism to grapple with the visual aspects of speech in relation to codes; systems afforded by visual language; rhetorics of visuality; and reading race, ethnicity, gender, sexuality, queerness, and economic class in the spaces and panels of the page.[6] That comics studies have rarely turned to theories of space as articulated in the philosophy of architecture and geography is both intriguing and an invitation to apply such approaches.[7] These philosophical, theoretical methodologies that focus on the built environment as impacted by and impacting the social invite a corollary to the spatial concerns of comics panels and framing. For panels are inhabited spaces whose imbricated meanings can be gleaned through Groensteen's spatio-topical comics system and Henri Lefebvre's philosophical socio-topical systems, the latter from his *The Production of Space.*

Comics panels are a communicative system according to Groensteen: "Pages situated opposite each other are dependent on a natural solidarity, and predisposed to speak to each other" (*System of Comics* 35). Panels' content and organization speak to each other, to readers, and project meaning among characters and icons. Comics for Groensteen are arthrologically structured or connected, from the Greek "arthron" meaning "articulation" (21), as referenced earlier in chapters on Davison's *The Spiral Cage* and Farmer's *Special Exits*. For the purposes of reading graphic pathography, I also reference the ability for "artho" to suggest "joint," an attribution to bodily connections. In the context of the multiframe—"the sum of the frames that compose a given comic"—comics forge meaning through interrelation, or through what Groensteen calls braiding (31, 21). While we read from start to finish and, in the Western world, from left to right, the spatio-topical system exercises readerly memory that remembers or reassembles out of "joint" icons, images, and sequences in order to build meaning, to work from the parts to the whole.

In *Comics and Narration*, Groensteen explores how comics rhythm is often interrupted by frames that defy the hegemony of an equally proportioned comics grid (what is often called a six-panel or nine-panel waffle grid). This disruption is a "felt" difference adjudicated by the reader and not related to how we might measure passing time through panel frequency or size (149). "The reader therefore contributes to the rhythm of the narration," Groensteen explains, "which, ultimately, coincides with the pulsating flow of the reading process" (151). A system of braided images across nonsequential frames and pages, combined with the reader's contributions to feeling or experiencing ruptured reading tempos, correlate affectively to theories about social spaces where tempered flows within them can be upset by surges of movement. The social spaces addressed by Marxist theorist Henri Lefebvre are necessarily "hypercomplex" because space is created by and consumes both energy and (human) bodies (93): "forces of production" are animated and enervated by class and labor (88, 90).[8] Lefebvre's philosophical-social argument in *The Production of Space* also advances a reticulated coherence, like Groensteen's spatio-topical comics system, here among mental, physical, intellectual, and social spaces in tension with each other. What we imagine or rationalize (mental space) cannot be separated from the concrete or physical (nature, the built environment), all of which inhere through the productive activity of social space (Lefebvre 36). For Lefebvre, space becomes or develops (into a house, an intersection, a park, a library) through accrued histories, especially related to power and its ability to ratify or refute subjects and agency (Lefebvre 110, 201). Waiting rooms are spaces fraught with power dynamics related to the homogeneity and hierarchy of medicine. When a comics waiting room is read through Groensteen's compositional system and Lefebvre's social space of production, it encompasses the physical, intellectual, and collective in the process of becoming lived and read space.

Those of Lefebvre's concepts that are related to authority—under which I consider medical knowledge, health care staff, pharmaceutical laboratories, and institutions of caring—find traction in graphic narratives, but in unexpected ways, especially in graphic pathography's powerful return of (or reply to) the medical gaze of authority in which the personal narrative looks (back) at the impersonal institution. Take this elaborate example from Marisa Acocella Marchetto's *Cancer Vixen* (a graphic pathography discussed in chapter 2) when autographic avatar Marisa repeatedly draws "actual size" renditions of a blood-drawing needle, a shot, and a chemo IV across her many cancer treatments (167). Readers who have not experienced and survived chemo, but only imagine its procedures, craft new relationships to the material objects of needles and IVs after reading her work. The medical implements that are depicted as life-sized on the page seem unduly enormous because readers are unused to seeing them as such in a comic. Their seemingly exaggerated depiction assists us in understanding Marisa's dread at each chemo session. Through actual-size representation, chemotherapy in *Cancer Vixen* can no longer serve as a mere linguistic term that noncancer subjects associate with cancer treatment. Rather, it reveals an action that is delivered, again and again, by the painful puncture from a series of sharp objects meant to inject or withdraw liquids. Marchetto's numeric accounting of her treatment needles—as in "needle #9" (161)—forges a framework of "needle-ness" that occurs only in the clinical space, uniting emotion (fear, anxiety) and anticipation with place. In fact, chemo patients often vomit before their scheduled treatment, so accustomed to the negative bodily reactions to the provided medicine.

Groensteen creates and defines needed comics-specific vocabulary for the field—such as multiframe, hyperframe, arthrology, braiding, among others—but says little about how they contribute to making meaning. Thus, turning to Lefebvre's critique of the mundane and the everyday as resistance to capitalism might productively steer comics criticism to consider what comics space means, for example, beyond sequential frames' depiction of chronological and nonchronological narratives. Graphic narrative's visual network of affiliated panels and repetitive symbols that draw out and upon Groensteen's spatio-topical system also recall Lefebvre's notion of the production of space, as the latter consists of waves, circuits, and networks. Both complex systems link parts to the whole as the production of meaning occurs across panels and pages in the former, through people, production, and power in the latter. Per sociologist Pierre Bourdieu, the culturally groomed behaviors we bring to the sociocultural (here medical) realm as well as capital we have attained or been denied (as raced or gendered individuals, for example, or in the form of available or nonexistent health insurance) play out among patients whose reactions to diagnoses or inability to pay for them might erupt in hidden or visible competitions. Hospital, clinic, and hospice waiting spaces resonate as habitats (dynamic surroundings, environments) and thus also reflect Bourdieu's habitus (for my purposes, accrued dispositions toward the culture of medicine).

Graphic pathography draws out the passing of time within and against the institutionalized time of waiting, diagnosis, prognosis, treatment, and remission. Disruptive authority in Lefebvre in relation to readers' reactions to disruptions of expected sequential monotony (as posited by Groensteen) assists me in exploring how comics criticism can pose questions about the culture of medicine and health through theories of spatial geography and approaches from the social sciences. What is brought to and circulates within the waiting room through social embodiment?[9] What happens to self- and other representation in that space?

Networks of Time, Space, and Culture

I examine four waiting rooms in this section, the first two preparatory examples. The latter delve deeply into comics' deliberative play through panels or splash pages, magnifying the circulating emotions of patients and their attending family members empaneled in comics waiting rooms. Near the middle of Judith Vanistendael's *When David Lost His Voice*, an aerial double-page spread captures character Paula and her daughter Tamar at a crossroads between the empty hallways of two hospital wings. A yellow-floored, wood-paneled corridor extends from the left of the book's gutter, exuding vitality and energy. This warm-hued hallway ushers healthy family members into the hospice ward, stretching to the right of the gutter, depicted in a clinical blue-green wash. Behind one of the doors in this second hallway lies David, Paula's husband and Tamar's father, dying from throat cancer.

Spots of crimson in Tamar's red hat and Paula's orange scarf contrast brightly against the light green walls and floor of the hospice ward. The contrast channels the notion of an energetic and lived diegetic past from which Paula and Tamar emerge before the lines of the horizontal hallway move our eyes into the antiseptic cancer wing, where David's future resides. Both hallways' hues bleed off the pages, an artistic suggestion of energy flowing within and through the institution, ushered in by patients, visitors, and the medical staff interacting with each other in various given and unexpected emotional states. In Paula's speech balloon, she instructs Tamar to "Wave your hand in front of the button" to activate the automatic door separating them from hospice, inviting them to bring their life into the subsequent place of demise (208). The location of the glassed-in alcove dividing the healthy from the ill serves literally as both the book's material gutter, the binding, and as a comics gutter, the space between two panels. Figuratively, mother and daughter are arrested by the portal, suspended between the world of the living and that of the dying.[10] Vanistendael's Paula, Tamar, and David are transient guests in the stable institution of the hospital; nobody stays there forever. Either David will walk out, or he will die and be carried out. Hospital doors, serving as gutters, interweave meanings attendant to clinical spatial arrangement to comics' strategic use of space. The two converge here when the desire for emotional connection (between David and his family members) meets clinical distancing.

Rachael Ball's graphic pathography *The Inflatable Woman* contains an aerial perspective of a hospital reception area, allowing the reader to watch protagonist Iris from above as she enters the hospital the morning of a check-up to assess two lumps discovered in one of her breasts (fig. 6). However, while Vanistendael's comics' corridor contributes to a sense of forward progression as its horizontal lines conduct our gaze from left to right, the narrow top-down shaft in Ball's graphic narrative telescopes readers into a tiny waiting room, confining our perspective and sense of movement. Like Iris, we feel trapped. The perspective drops us into the cell-like space from the wide expanse above, an artistic maneuver that channels Iris's growing anxiety. For Elisabeth El Refaie, depicting a character "from a high angle and a great distance" contributes to the sense of vulnerability the artist intends to convey (7).[11] The windowpanes of the French doors on opposite sides of the room mimic the square cubbies behind the receptionist. Despite the order provided by these metrical squares, their uniformity is more haunting than reassuring, their emptiness (including unadorned walls and blank sheet of notepaper) is eerily vacant for such a full-bodied experience, while the narrowing of perspective becomes stifling.

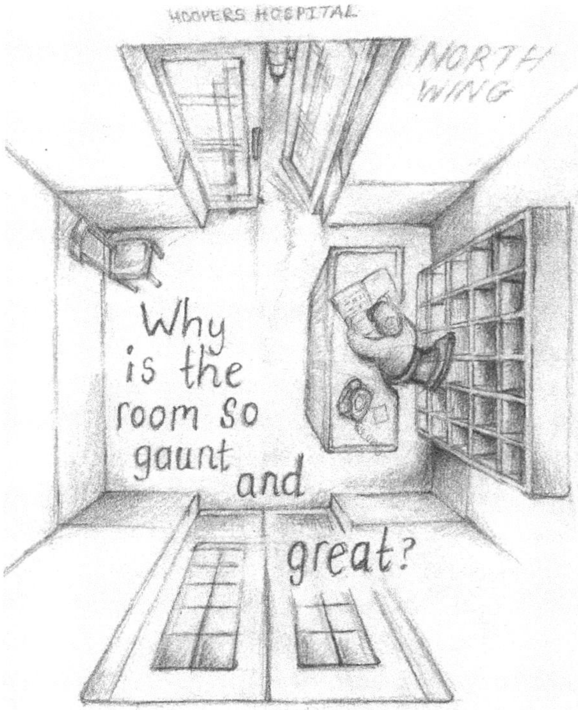

Fig. 6 | An anxiety-producing perspective of the cell-like reception area of the hospital before Iris's mastectomy. From Rachael Ball, *The Inflatable Woman*, 2015, p. 36. Courtesy of Rachael Ball.

In his *Graphic Storytelling and Visual Narrative*, Will Eisner theorizes that a view from above presents perspectival advantage for reader and characters who might be doing the looking, especially when positioned above a potential threat (in Eisner's case, a monster-like figure).[12] They see the threat from on high; it cannot see them unless prompted to look up, an unlikely scenario if the subject hopes to quietly conceal herself from the monster. In contrast, a view originating from below is more ominous, as Eisner's monster, with an effortless glance down, might notice the frightened character. The top-down perspective in *The Inflatable Woman* plunges us from an expanse above into the oppressive confines of the cell-like waiting room of Hooper's Hospital, depicted as a cold, lonely, and frightening environment. One hard, wooden chair sits empty in a corner; a reception desk two paces away is staffed by a woman, the only other person in the room, preoccupied by reading a book. The words "Why is the room so gaunt and great?" take up much space across the empty floor and scroll onto the canted windows of one of the walls (36). The page's single panel captures Iris's feelings of intense apprehension and lack of control. Graphic pathography participates in such visual constructs and perspectives, creatively visioning the mood and tone of accepted constructs like the waiting room through new eyes.

Discerned dispositions and intuited temperaments augment the already cramped quarters of a tidy visitors' corner adjacent to a surgical unit in Ware's *Jimmy Corrigan*. It contrasts starkly with the busy, sprawling patients' lounge in the infertility clinic of Potts's *Good Eggs*. While compositionally at odds—one ordered, the other chaotic—they both promote graphic empathy in their illustrated critique of medical time and space. In *Jimmy Corrigan*, protagonist Jimmy is a white, middle-aged, unmarried, assumedly cisgendered, and unattached man, generally fearful of people, events, and places beyond the perceived safety of home and work. While hundreds of Jimmy-featured images appear in the graphic narrative's panels, the character does little to nothing within them. He is a passive subject waiting to be acted upon. Emotionally reclusive, socially awkward, uninterested in much, he seems unlike "the smartest kid on earth" of the graphic narrative's subtitle. In contrast to Jimmy's banality is the comics' compositionally paradoxical gridding: Ware never draws the same layout twice over a three-hundred-and-fifty-page narrative. The busy reticulated pages, consisting of ruler-straight black frames in an endless array of sizes and configurations, proffer an incessant variation starkly at odds with Jimmy's singular, monotonous response—anxiety—to the world around him. Because Jimmy is controlled by his environments, subjected to authorities (per Lefebvre)—such as his father, the narrative's doctor, his sister, all of whom he diligently obeys—I argue that Ware's space inhabits Jimmy; Jimmy does not command his own place.[13]

Contrasted to Ware's ramrod gridding are Potts's messier, hand-drawn frames. *Good Eggs* charts the infertility protocol of her white autographic protagonist Phoebe and her white husband Jeff, a step-by-step personal and medical process requiring precise attention to time, to Phoebe's menstrual cycles. Her squiggly lines and textured images, appearing both in hand-drawn grids and as free-floating characters on unpaneled pages, depict the systemic and often chaotic, but not always effective, in vitro fertilization. The human body's fluctuating inconsistencies, the images project, can trip up a methodical, scientific procedure. Phoebe is brought closer to her husband Jeff because of their inability to conceive; they talk, hug, hold hands, attend events together in many of the panels, suggesting not only their affection for each other but also their understanding that the infertility challenge is a mutual responsibility.

Intimacy is starkly absent in *Jimmy Corrigan*. Jimmy is estranged from his father and unaware of the existence of his sister until the siblings meet in the ER over James Corrigan's (or Jimmy Sr.'s) accident. The siblings are closely related by blood, but distant for never meeting until they become adults. For Jimmy, the siblings also are visibly and uncomfortably separated by race. Amy is an adopted African American child; unknown to the contemporary Corrigan family, Amy has descended from Jimmy's great-grandfather's sexual liaison, most likely by sexual violation of his black maid.[14] The family's history is associated with violence and desertion,[15] not love or intimacy, the latter into which the siblings are forced in the alarmingly small space of the hospital's emergency waiting room, knee to knee, a gutter between them.[16] In Kate Polak's *Ethics in the Gutter*, she regards this comics element "more as a space that creates the 'room' to imagine connections" (1). Ware's space gives us room to connect race in the past and the present of the Corrigans' worlds, discussed more at length below. Because both characters choose silence over engaging in unnecessary chatter, it is only the awkward sounds of "scrnch" and schooch" emitted when they sit down or shift on plastic seats that fill the quiet space with sound. In a graphic narrative about a bumbling, socially inept protagonist, the extra "SSSsss" exhaling from his seat cushion gives him the last, embarrassing "word" before the two settle into their awkward uncommunicativeness.

Mr. Corrigan is the familial figure that genetically knits together Amy and Jimmy, whose long separation from each other, given the family's inability to remain united, becomes uncomfortably pronounced in the ER waiting room. They are physically close in the cramped space, but not affectionately close. Amy arrives at the hospital before she hears of her father's passing, bearing a clean set of his clothing, including, wishfully, a pair of his tennis shoes (fig. 7). Meanwhile, Jimmy arrives hobbled by a crutch, one foot bound in a white bandage, after being clipped by a car. Ironically, beyond connection by family association, injury to his foot correlates him materially to Amy, the wistful bearer of shoes, and to his father by bodily harm, the latter (fatally) injured in a different car accident. That both men will never wear the shoes dissociates Jimmy from his half-sister. After hearing the news of Mr. Corrigan's death, Amy's hand trembles in rage. She finally pushes Jimmy to the floor, lowering him in her own estimation and to Jimmy's already pathetic low self-estimation. The graphic narrative concludes with the intimation that Amy and Jimmy have permanently separated after this brief, unhappy union. They will remain silent siblings to each other, without further contact following their brief intimacy, knee to knee, in the cramped ER waiting room.[17]

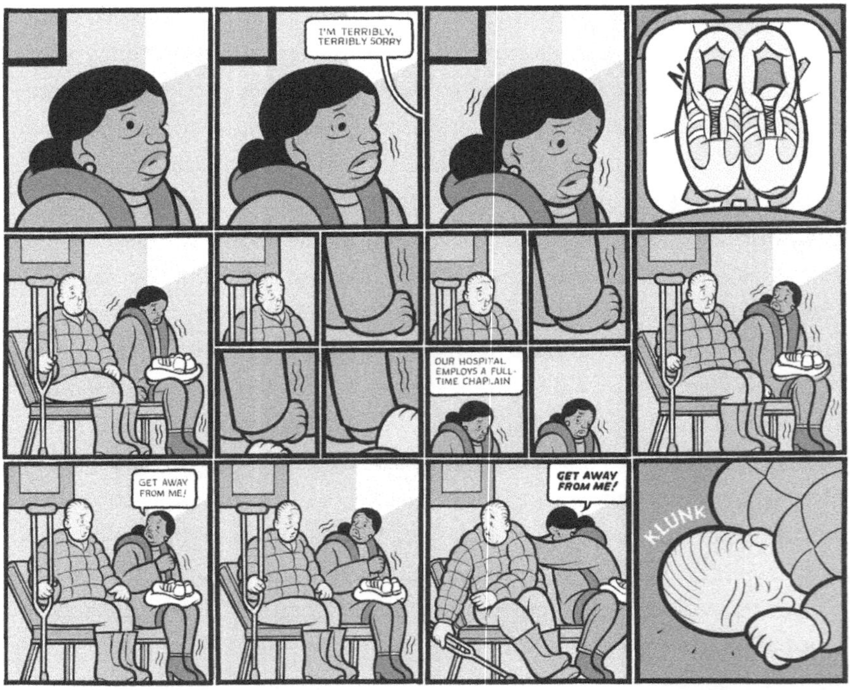
I'M TERRIBLY, TERRIBLY SORRY
OUR HOSPITAL EMPLOYS A FULL-TIME CHAPLAIN
GET AWAY FROM ME!
GET AWAY FROM ME!
KLUNK

Fig. 7 | Amy shoves Jimmy off the bench. From Chris Ware, *Jimmy Corrigan: The Smartest Kid on Earth*, 2003, n.p. Courtesy of Chris Ware.

Color in Ware's waiting-room space is connected with readings about race.[18] Ware's color scheme creates a chromatic harmony that immediately contradicts the racial disharmony Amy has experienced and expects from those who are unfamiliar with the fact that, as adopted, she is not supposed to be biologically related to white James Corrigan, yet her ancestry (ushering from a sexual violation of a black maid by Jimmy's great-great grandfather) reveals the fascinating ways in which one generation's actions return to impact that of another. A two-seated couch in tangerine orange sits beneath a reproduction of Paul Cézanne's peaches.[19] The orange color of both the bench and painting are congenially matched. Meanwhile, hospital personnel's confusion over (white) Mr. Corrigan's paternity to (black) daughter Amy Corrigan—each not of the same "color"—is exacerbated because the ward is releasing a black patient also named "Mr. Corrigan." Clearly, Ware's inclusion of this unlikely coincidence is a play on our assumptions about race, genealogy, and inheritance. Furthermore, Amy's pink jacket and blue jeans juxtaposed against the orange seat manufacture a compendium dissonance mirroring the confusion over race relations (by way of color) in this scene of multiply "colored" Corrigans. As some of the most brightly hued panels in the narrative—in which orange and pink might be described as "warm"—it is ironic that the occasion incites racial misrecognition and strife.

National racial discourses, sedimented through history, have "oriented" Amy's black body toward the care of others. By sedimentation I mean social expectations held by nonblack subjects toward black subjects, like the stereotypical, corporeal mammy whose fleshy body was physically and metaphorically regarded as capacious enough to embody (care for) her own and her white mistress's children. I also mean the sedimentation of history in that Mammy becomes the center of the black household, the woman in whom the black family historically has been grounded, then blamed for destroying the patriarchal family if the black paternal head of household departs. Representation is thus stuck in a racist, hierarchical or stacked past, socially disciplining Amy into avenues of ministration. In their "Graphic Whiteness and the Lessons of Chris Ware's *Jimmy Corrigan*," Juda Bennett and Cassandra Jackson argue that when Amy, herself a nurse, tends to one of Jimmy's wounds from a former mishap, "Ware further emphasizes their roles as racially defined and positions Amy problematically as caretaker to white brokenness" (n.p.). Furthermore, they argue, Amy's presence is geared toward "healing, or at least to explaining, ancestral history. Blackness, in other words, serves to heal, explain, or justify whiteness" (n.p.). We are aware that black women have a history of caring for black and white men throughout slavery, into its aftermath, and to the present day, afflicted by undue responsibility. We might thus surmise that Amy has been caring for her father. First left by her biological parents for adoption, then assuming care of her father and seemingly of her invalid brother Jimmy, she is understandably enraged at what might feel like a cascade of unwieldy responsibility sedimented by a racist history. Her understanding is thus: during Jimmy's twenty-four-hour visit at his father's house, and after a thirty-or-more-year separation, her father is hospitalized and dies; meanwhile, for years under Amy's watchful, daughterly care, James thrived.

Ware's paneling in the figure above pairs the siblings visually and suggests accord, as in the second and third rows where the characters remain seated next to each other, each equally represented. The first panel of the series depicts only Amy's head and shoulders, the last only Jimmy's as he lies on the ground. In between, Amy holds a *pair* of her father's white shoes and a white T-shirt, the former intimating the possibility of sibling affinity (or pairing) despite years of being unaware of the other's existence. That

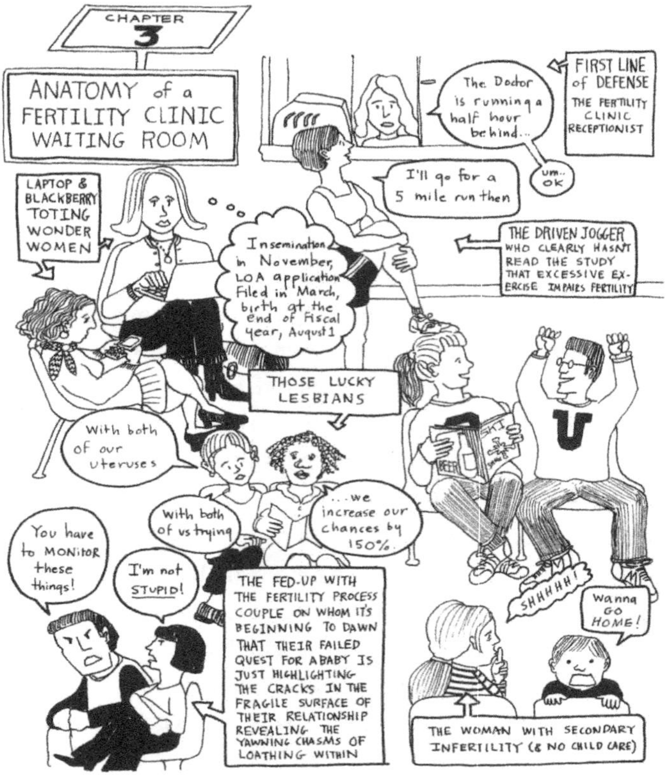
CHAPTER 3
ANATOMY of a FERTILITY CLINIC WAITING ROOM
The Doctor is running a half hour behind...
FIRST LINE of DEFENSE THE FERTILITY CLINIC RECEPTIONIST
I'll go for a 5 mile run then
um.. ok
LAPTOP & BLACKBERRY TOTING WONDER WOMEN
Insemination in November, LOA application Filed in March, birth at the end of Fiscal year, August 1
THE DRIVEN JOGGER WHO CLEARLY HASN'T READ THE STUDY THAT EXCESSIVE EXERCISE IMPAIRS FERTILITY
THOSE LUCKY LESBIANS
With both of our uteruses
With both of us trying
...we increase our chances by 150%.
You have to MONITOR these things!
I'm not STUPID!
THE FED-UP WITH THE FERTILITY PROCESS COUPLE ON WHOM IT'S BEGINNING TO DAWN THAT THEIR FAILED QUEST FOR A BABY IS JUST HIGHLIGHTING THE CRACKS IN THE FRAGILE SURFACE OF THEIR RELATIONSHIP REVEALING THE YAWNING CHASMS OF LOATHING WITHIN
SHHHHH!
Wanna GO HOME!
THE WOMAN WITH SECONDARY INFERTILITY (& NO CHILD CARE)

Amy, the adopted daughter, not Jimmy, the biological son, holds remnants of paternity endows her with a white lineage often denied mixed-race bodies. The lustrous blanched shoes and T-shirt are uncannily centralized by their vibrancy. The items also are accorded an important, upper-right-hand panel, a standard stopping place for the eye in Western reading practice before it moves left and down to the next line. After a close-up, however, in which the white items inhabit most of the frame, they recede but do not disappear because their luminescence cannot be ignored among the panels' other bright colors. One black and one white sibling cannot amiably consolidate in their grief, implying how the narrative and the siblings are racially charged and how that charge subtly infiltrates their waiting space.

Ware's tightly paneled ER nook contrasts sharply with Potts's completely free-form double-page spread "Anatomy of a Fertility Clinic Waiting Room" (98–99) (figs. 8 and 9). Nearly every blank space is occupied by images, speech balloons, clinic signage, and Potts's captions. Unlike the strictly dictated reading order prescribed by Ware's panel structure, readers wander across

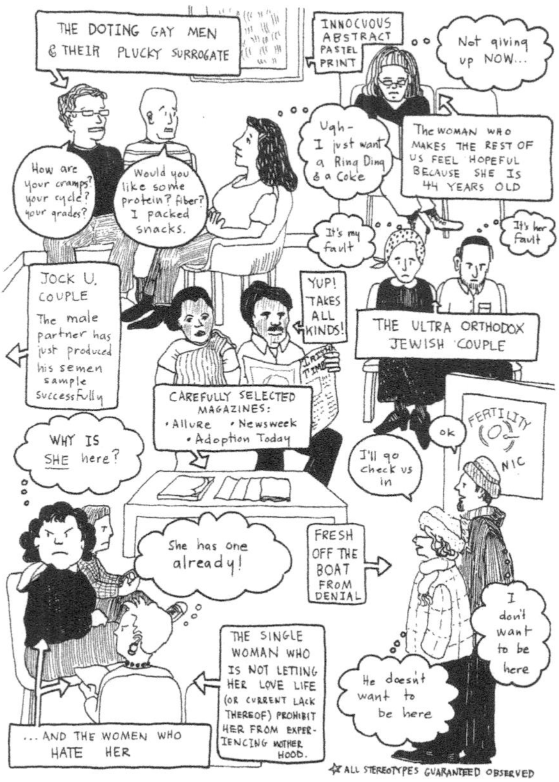

Fig. 8 | While waiting intimates passivity, the dynamism of Potts's spread is palpable. From *Good Eggs* by Phoebe Potts, pp. 98–99. Copyright © 2010 by Phoebe Potts. Used by permission of HarperCollins Publishers.

Potts's two linked pages horizontally, left to right, or right to left, or even vertically and then horizontally. Beyond being arrested by a single centralized image of a young couple, addressed below, no correct reading pattern is required to understand the scene. Any reading approach will convey this upshot: infertility treatments are not guaranteed to work, they are anxiety producing, and they often silently pit patients against each other. Chinmay Murali and Sathyaraj Venkatesan claim that Potts's "narrative demonstrates the cultural valorisation of childrearing, which would inevitably ostracise the childless," played out here in the competitive encounter of the waiting room (*Infertility Comics and Graphic Medicine* 60).[20]

While waiting intimates passivity, the dynamism of Potts's spread is palpable. Gesticulating, whining, angry, and frustrated characters energize the wait. Their conversations and body postures reveal their emotions. We can see the patients' full bodies in contrast to only the head and neck of an administrative assistant behind a sliding glass window and the partial view of an infertility specialist who, in later panels, is shielded by a desk and computer while discussing Phoebe and Jeff's infertility situation. As he informs them about procedures, his speech balloon takes up three-quarters of the panel, yet much of what he is explaining is indecipherable. Potts thus denotes a bewildering amount of technical information confronting overwhelmed Phoebe and Jeff through their puzzled "Huh?" and an "Um . . ." (103). They are reduced to uttering linguistic fillers against the specialist's cryptic messages, each talking past the other.

Class, culture, and social standing contribute to what we bring to a space and how we shape and are shaped by it. For example, reproducing (having children) in American national culture is power. Giving birth to a biological child is forward thinking[21]—one recreates, regenerates, and brings progeny into the present for the future. It invites entrance into formal lineage, the line (forward) inextricably associated with the past through heritage and genealogy. For Phoebe and Jeff, however, one of the two carries a genealogical past that prevents that phenomenon, driving them (whether forward or backward is for the reader to decide) to experts. In *Kimiko Does Cancer*, by Keet Geniza (artist) and Kimiko Tobimatsu (author, contributor), the walls of the fertility clinic where protagonist Kimiko harvests and freezes her eggs before breast cancer surgery are lined with pictures of cute babies, all staring adorably from their frames at the reader, positioned above waiting patients who are "all older [than twenty-five-year-old Kimiko] and desperate to be parents" (24). This choice of wall decoration seems intentionally cruel for the childless and the infertile.

Phoebe's captions iterate her understanding of the positions and status of patients in waiting, many seemingly culturally disempowered by infertility. Potts's drawn arrow pointing to what she captions as an "innocuous abstract pastel print" behind her implies the neutrality this waiting room is to exude: abstracts invite a variety of interpretations that cannot be proved wrong (99). In contrast, the women perturbed by another who is quieting her noisy child alters that proposed neutrality with resentment: she has a child, and they do not, their reactions intone. Positioned in the bottom right-hand corner of the spread are Phoebe and Jeff whose thought bubbles echo each other, from Phoebe's "He doesn't want to be here" to Jeff's "I don't want to be here" (99).

Potts's arrangement in the waiting room's double-page spread visually favors a young white couple in sweatshirts bearing what seem like university logos. Potts aptly, then, captions them the "Jock U Couple" (98). They exhibit clear camaraderie, comfortable in their bodies and in the situation, possessing the advantages of being white, young, and college educated. The young man of the duo raises his fists in victory over having "just produced his semen sample successfully" (98). In addition to their prime space near the center of the double-page spread, generous white space surrounding them visually highlights this aesthetically manufactured prominence. Potts's framing connotes that white, educated, heterosexual youths of the page's visual spotlight (or even as its highlight) epitomize our future and our strength (remember the man's raised fist over his successful ejaculation).

The disorganization of Potts's representative waiting space chafes against the assumed order of science in clinical care, where facts, theories, and experimentation presuppose linearity and positivism. The field of the health humanities, in contrast, claims that the narrative nature of medicine, more akin to social and cultural constructions than scientific determinations, might more rightfully claim medicine as both science and art.[22] Interpretations are not accepted truths; patients often turn to a second *opinion*, as diagnoses are clinical judgments, defined by Kathryn Montgomery in her *How Doctors Think* (32): "Because clinicians are immersed in unpredictable circumstances, they often must respond experimentally, using their best guesses and watching for confirmation or failure" (59).

Inconsistencies and gaps remain fundamental elements of a profession steeped in knowledge and hermeneutics that undergird the hopes and fears circulating in hospital waiting rooms. Imbricated sociocultural spaces in Ware's and Potts's waiting arenas emphasize how the profound existence of ambiguity—as when patients inquire, Will I live through cancer? Will I have children? Will I recover?—affects, or shapes, cultural spaces. In this study's conclusion, I argue for the necessity of ambiguity. The next chapter, however, takes up a profound and deleterious gap in graphic pathography—that of representations of race. I examine disease, disability, wounding, and the myth of the model minority through the impending blindness of an Asian North American character.

Chapter 5

Graphting and the Model Minority in Chong and Webber's *Dancing After TEN*

James Kyung-Jin Lee argues that although illness memoirs by Asian North Americans have arrived late to the burgeoning genre, their contemporary consumption is not only "most important" but also "possibly most treacherous" (16).[1] In his *Pedagogies of Woundedness: Illness, Memoir, and the Ends of the Model Minority*, ill or incapacitated Asian North American doctor-subjects contend with both the embodied cost of illness and its consequences to their model minority status. While the latter is not of their own making, the myth has provided them a smoother path, compared to other minorities, to national acceptance, even financial solidity, despite the fact that—or because—they are tethered to this elevating but problematic cultural narrative. When Asian North American physicians experience disease or impairment, their minority narrative is "wrecked," Lee argues (quoting Arthur Frank 16). The arduous ascent to a "better present" in a racist world seems for naught when incapacitation eclipses anticipated further model minority advancement (17). The myth has schooled them to be strong, persistent, and productive. When too ill to carry out its expectations, they self-regard as failures while continuing to uphold its fictions. It is not the decline in bodily health that should be detrimental, argues Lee, but rather the "deeply toxic dimensions" (21) of "a disciplined, healthy body that mirrors the socially and economic productive life" laid out in the myth (20). The narrative functions complementarily and perniciously at once. In this chapter, I explore how the racial category "Asian North American" functions within, then beyond, the wounding aspects and expectations of the model minority in Vivian Chong and Georgia Webber's *Dancing After TEN*.[2]

Lee, who has built his scholarly reputation in Asian North American studies and race and ethnic studies, fully grasps the intricacies and tensions between race and health. In the wider field of disability studies, intersectional approaches appear as possible anti-essentialist solutions to persistent challenges of representation, but often without clear indication of subjects' racial identification. Identity categories are "mutually interdependent," argue Tina Goethals, Elisabeth De Schauwer, and Geert Van Hove on the necessity of "weaving" intersectionality into disability studies in the research (75). To remedy this dearth of references to race and structural inequality in the field, I turn to Chris Bell, both later in this chapter and in the coda, who laments the whiteness of the field in "Introducing White Disability Studies: A Modest Proposal" and in his edited collection *Blackness and Disability*. They constitute initial necessary considerations of race in the disability studies arena.[3] I ask, if clinical medicine has relied on white men subjects as standard bearers in testing, how does an Asian North American's self-representation in comics change how we see the category Asian and model minority?

In brief summary, *Dancing After TEN* charts graphic designer Vivian Chong's journey into blindness. In 2004, she lost most of her eyesight to toxic epidermal necrolysis syndrome (TEN) after an extremely rare reaction to ibuprofen. Patients afflicted by this condition might experience skin lesions that scar organs such as the eyeball and eardrum, eventually affecting sight and hearing. TEN might cause hemorrhaging and respiratory failure, and can result in death. Before being blinded by TEN-related corneal scar tissue, she solicited artist Georgia Webber to collaborate on what eventually became the graphic memoir *Dancing After TEN*. With artistic contributions from both Chong and Webber, the graphic pathography charts the former's journey before, during, and after contracting TEN. Chong partners with Webber because she, too, experienced sensory diminishment, albeit not permanent, as is Wong's blindness. For a substantial period, Webber lost her voice, subsequently her job, some of her friends, and fell into depression. She chronicles this period of voicelessness and anxiety in her graphic memoir *Dumb: Living Without a Voice*. In *Dancing After TEN*, when Chong can no longer see well enough to craft a recognizable, representative self, Webber draws Chong's comics under Wong's explicit verbal direction.[4] What Chong remembers is given legible "voice" through Webber's hand.

Dancing After TEN, I argue throughout, is graphic pathography against clinical and race determinations, a necessary extrication from expectation. To be recognized as Asian Canadian or Asian North American, terms I use interchangeably despite some historical differences between Canadian and American immigration laws pertaining to Asians, is an evolving distinction based on the relevance of race to the vagaries of society and politics. Because the racial, biological markers of Asian North Americans resist invisibility (almond-shaped and dark eyes, black hair), and because Asian North Americans proudly embrace their race and ethnicity as aspects of their humanity, ignoring racial identity is injurious. Color blindness is one such attempt, unsuccessful in that the term itself asserts the existence of color before ironically declaring color/race's invisibility. Even when Vivian is seemingly overlooked as an Asian Canadian, specifically when her (almond-shaped) eyes are obscured behind dark sunglasses, my reading magnifies how minimizing references to race in the graphic narrative is deleterious to Vivian's and *TEN*'s readers. *Dancing After TEN* is Chong's bold challenge to model minority expectations levied against Asian North Americans, in sickness and in health. In drawing her woundedness, Wong manages her self-depiction.

Dancing After TEN also interrogates Chong's nonhierarchical collaboration with Webber. The equitable partnership grates against past artistic comics partnerships among white subjects in which a stratification reigns in graphic narratives authored and illustrated by two people: the author is listed on the cover first, the artist second (although this is not true in European graphic narrative). Chong and Webber both as subjects of impairment, permanent and temporary respectively, learn from each other in an innovative, nonhierarchical transmission I call graphting—a suturing and a regeneration—which I define carefully later in the chapter. The two cooperatively delineate loss and draw against self-dispossession and impairment.

Graphic Pathography Collaborations

In this section, I compare and contrast previously published collaborative autobiographical graphic narratives to Chong and Webber's joint creation. *Dancing After TEN* is innovatively distinct from others on the market. First, because the artists depend on each other's unique abilities and symbiotic understanding of disability: blindness for Chong and temporary voicelessness for Webber; second because the graphic narrative extends discussions of how race matters in publishing, a topic inadequately addressed in graphic pathography.

Collaboration is an established feature of superhero comics, long a staple in the comics field. The shared labor consists of authors who create the storyline, artists who draw the images, and those who ink, letter, and produce the entire look of each page. The many-handed partnership, however, challenges ownership over the final work that an autography need rarely address in our common understanding of the one-to-one correspondence between "auto" and "self." Yet for comics artist Harvey Pekar, he freely surrendered the artistic creation of "his" autobiographical self in *American Splendor* to graphic artists, including, but not limited to, Alison Bechdel, Robert Crumb, Joe Sacco, and Alan Moore. Notwithstanding contributions by such well-known artists, it is through Pekar's (authorial) fame and name that we reference *American Splendor*, not those of his (artist) comics biographers. The seventeen-issue series written by Pekar and illustrated by handpicked cartoonists was published from 1976 to 2008, charting avatar Harvey's pedestrian life as a white, middle-class, heterosexual man employed in a Cleveland Ohio–based Veterans Affairs office. The series illustrates his chats with friends, dashes to the bakery, to the dry cleaners, among other mundane activities. Collaborators were invited to depict character Harvey in their own distinctive drawing styles, emphasizing various aspects of the protagonist based on their subjective observations and individual interactions with him.

The series was revolutionary not only because of its unique collaboration, in which an autobiography was not drawn by the artist himself,[5] but also because it elevated depictions of ordinary life to the level of the exceptional—American splendor indeed. Thomas Bredehoft alleges that in *American Splendor*, Pekar maintained "an important degree of control over the artwork" (as a kind of "casting director" [102]), but what profoundly puzzles Bredehoft is that Carole Sobocinski, one of Pekar's chosen artists, employs an Art-Spiegelman-like hand, a *Maus*-ness, in *Splendor*'s chapter "The Man Who Came to Dinner—and Lunch and Breakfast" (100, 101).[6] On the one hand, it suggests that Pekar permitted a variety of unrepresentative (self-) images to evoke his likeness. On the other, it strikes a chord of extreme discomfort that Spiegelman's references to the Holocaust in *Maus I* and *II* are repurposed in *American Splendor* to animate Harvey's workaday, nonthreatened, nontraumatic life (Pekar was raised by Polish Jews who immigrated to the United States[7]). His approval of a *Maus*-ish Harvey demonstrates the strange paradox of Pekar's desire to represent the common, middle-class, American man delineated through Spegielman's terrorized mice.

Chong, however, who rapidly sketched her experiences journeying *into* blindness *as* blindness encroached, requested that Webber's style match her own as closely as possible.[8] Unlike *American Splendor* in which various distinctive approaches result in artistically symptomatic depictions of character Harvey, Webber's hand is less palimpsestic than hybridized. If the artistic style of an autographic forges a personal relation to content, Chong's emotional and psychological experiences of being hospitalized, incrementally losing her sight, living as an unsighted person, and handing over her self-representation to Webber require that the artists work in close cooperation. This contrasts with Pekar's seeming casual indifference to others' depictions of him. Chong was adamant about preserving, as much as possible, some semblance to her own artistic style. Through extensive and frequent phone and email communication, Webber spent countless hours explaining and narrating how her images epitomized Chong's own vision of protagonist Vivian. Webber committed an equally enormous amount of attention to incorporating Chong's feedback for final edits and approvals. The collaboration and a looming imposing deadline were so exhausting that Webber fell ill briefly.

Because featuring the prosaic routines of an average so-called everyman had never been committed to graphic memoir before, *American Splendor* was deemed exceptionally unique. Pekar's willingness to cede to others self-representations of his pedestrian life was a calculated but successful risk. In contrast, Chong and Webber chart the atypical and traumatic: that of the encroaching blindness of a graphic designer whose profession and livelihood depend on sight. Furthermore, Pekar's *American Splendor* as an outstanding innovation of an undistinguished office clerk chafes against the less generous denotation of how the blind stand out: they can be conspicuous through reliance on a red-and-white cane, sunglasses worn indoors, and perhaps a guide dog. Pekar's serialized innovation was further boosted through privileges granted by the publishing industry to a healthy white (ethnically Jewish) man: the unremarkable life of a common man deserved publication while his collaborators seemed delighted to spend countless hours drawing Harvey immersed in daily routines. When arrested by a bout of cancer, documented in union with his partner Joyce Brabner in the graphic narrative *Our Cancer Year* (illustrated by Frank Stack) and which I do not discuss in detail here, the notoriety accrued from *American Splendor* shepherded subsequent interest in this cancer memoir.

Asian North Americans, no matter the mundanity of their lives, typically have been exceptionalized by their race as "aliens" or robotic model minorities. Asian North Americans have been represented over time by others' caricatures of them rather than through self-representation. Jeff Yang and D. Daniel Kim collect and display a history of Asian caricature influenced by American anti-Asian sentiment and politics: early twentieth-century American publications featured Fu Manchu, Dragon Ladies, and Charlie Chan, among other Chinese types that were rehearsed in their 2011 curated exhibit *Marvels and Monsters: Unmasking Asian Images in U.S. Comics, 1942–1986* at New York University's Fales Library and Special Collections.[9] Chinese immigrants and Asian North Americans are differentiated from non-Asian populations through their eyes, hair, and often, but not always, their skin color. It marks them for a different kind of distinction than that which Pekar enjoys. The former encounter discrimination, are upheld troublingly as model minorities, or rendered politically invisible, all of which can impact them psychically and emotionally. In *Dancing After TEN*, Vivian relearns how to attend to circadian rhythms as a blind person in mainstream society and as a subject whose race is an exception to the norms of whiteness; in fact, completing the graphic narrative is more remarkable than not. Her daily challenges surpass Harvey's simple circulation in the world as a healthy man; her publication challenges are circumscribed by how race gets written on the page.

Race on the White, So-Called Blank Page

Race provides potentially significant venues for deepening and widening approaches to the field of graphic medicine. Health care and the health humanities, both of which oversee human flesh (literally and metaphorically), often also overlook specific needs of nonwhite patients, or append the results of drug trials executed on white bodies to all raced bodies, at disproportionate injury to patients of color. Acknowledging the life of race in clinical medicine and the cultural representation of Asian Americans over time are significant to my arguments about the Asian North American marked body in history. I therefore am compelled to excavate the muted presence of race in *Dancing After TEN*. The coda, "The Absent Presence of Race," explores continued and disturbing instances in which white artists' experiences of illness are universalized for all subjects in the health care system and on the comics page.

The whiteness of graphic medicine harmfully suggests that black, Asian, and Latinx bodies are healthy and able bodied. This allows culturally constructed, stereotyped narratives about race to take precedence in the rare appearances of impaired subjects of color, states Christopher Bell ("Introduction" 3). His work aims to "deconstruct the systems that would keep these bodies in separate spheres" (3). Borrowing from Bell, I perform "recovery work" on the bodies of color left out of disability studies (3). And from James Kyung-Jin Lee's argument, I attend to Asian North Americans' wounded bodies afflicted by diseases that might affect all humans and those debilitated by culturally constricting narratives crafted around their race.

Under the auspices of biopower (white) patients are diagnosed, or narrativized, by (white) doctors; in graphic pathography, such (white) patients craft views that more accurately capture how they image and narrate themselves. I parenthetically emphasize white patients and white health care providers, elucidating that, typically, racially unmarked subjects in graphic narrative are deemed white, hence universal. To foreground a nonwhite character's race is to remove them from this accepted and acceptable white universality. Only white people are rewarded recognition as "only" or uniquely people.[10] As the standard bearers of general (accepted, easily recognized) personhood, deviations through illustrated skin shading, hair type, and eye shape negatively mark race as the "not" white, the different, or the other against this standard.

In *Dancing After TEN*, Chong is Chinese Canadian, Webber white, yet Vivian's depictions provide scant evidence of her race. On the one hand, the absence of race on the page of a comic by an author named "Chong" prompts a preoccupation with reading for race. What occurs when Vivian's race is not in plain sight, to borrow the title of Ralph Rodriguez's essay about the "racial surfaces" of graphic narratives by Japanese American cartoonist Adrian Tomine (102)? And what happens when "'reading' fails," asks Olivia Banner in exploring the consequences of nonwhite characters' white passing (34)? When we animate racial meanings from our own assumptions (from character to caricature, for example), we may commit a disservice to the text itself, Rodriguez explains. He eschews this kind of "symptomatic reading," one defined by Stephen Best and Sharon Marcus (89). They argue that symptomatic reading deliberately searches for, and ultimately finds, what it seeks in a text's gaps and absences. Such a "paranoid" reading process, a term initially employed by Eve Kosovsky Sedgwick, is one that always reads race into content, even when the content might not support such a reading (Rodriguez 92). Against Rodriguez's advice, I avoid literary paranoia by rendering race meaningful, sometimes paradoxical, in *TEN*'s rare representations of race.

In fact, it is quite paradoxical that Vivian's Asianness, most evident in the almond shape of her eyes, disappears behind her sunglasses, for it is her physical, visible eye shape that has made discernible the Asian aspect of her

Asian Canadian identity. Chong dedicates the book to these eyes that readers of her work do not see: "You have gone through so much . . . [but] 'Eyes,' you still are beautiful" (n.p.). That is, these self-defined beautiful Asian eyes are tucked behind Chong's sunglasses in her photograph on the dedication page, but the prose suggests that beauty, here, is not in the contours of her Asian eyes but in their valuable contributions to her "aesthetic sensibility" (*TEN*'s Dedication n.p.). She feels and remembers her way to beauty as corporeal resonance, even though eventually she cannot see her own beauty. Society defines her race through the shape of her eyes, while Vivian defines the creative shape of her imagination through what her eyes once beheld. In the paratext of *Dancing After TEN*, biographical material about artists Chong and Webber forgoes the following information easily found online: Chong was born in Hong Kong and later immigrated to Toronto. This omission aligns with the graphic narrative's seemingly unconscious erasure of Vivian's corporeal race signifiers. Only through reference to Vivian's Chinese mother in the first half of the graphic narrative are we introduced to her racial heritage. The following addresses how we might reconstitute, or see, a raced body through the hand (drawings) of a raced subject who can no longer see.

Race functions as a symptom for investigative diagnosis. The cover of *Dancing After TEN* denotes the book "a graphic memoir." If we know nothing about its contents, the cover suggests that it is the autobiography of a woman—either the "Chong" or "Webber" listed there—perhaps traumatized by an ailment affecting her physical ability. The artists' names are printed beneath a woman's form shifting iteratively by stages from crouching to standing to dancing. The surname "Chong" implies an Asian North American author; the surname "Webber" that follows it denotes an Anglo-Saxon one. We are compelled to ask, whose memoir is this?[11]

The narrative's opening spread also offers no clues to the identity of the protagonist. If we eventually understand that on the memoir's first page the woman in sunglasses sitting in a WestJet gate with a suitcase at her knee is blind Vivian, we might find it cruel that the unidentified man rolling a suitcase of his own asks of her, in the manner of a traveling companion and not a stranger, "I'm going to get a coke. Watch my bag, okay?" (1). This introduction to Vivian and an ex-boyfriend who agrees to accompany her to an eye operation signifies how assumptions about seeing and being seen work in two ways, literally and metaphorically: first, if she is blind, she cannot watch Seth's bag. Second, wearing dark glasses at the gate relates to how the "hieroglyphs" of Asian Canadian identity, as defined by Eleanor Ty, can be both visible and hidden (*Politics of the Visible* 3).[12] Vivian's racial designation as Asian Canadian, distinctly through the shape of her eyes, is eclipsed by dark glasses. As a typically identifiable Asian Canadian, Vivian in sunglasses is now less visibly distinct from non-Asian Canadians. Racial markings are exceptions to the rule of whiteness, historically contributing to how Chinese immigrants to both Canada and the United States faced racist laws and social discrimination and how anti-Asian sentiment played out during the COVID-19 pandemic as violence against Asian subjects. Or in Lee's iteration of Asian North Americans and race, to be regarded as cultural emblems of success through the myth of the model minority is wounding by turns, tamping expected ascendancy of those Asian North Americans who fall ill and assuming the self-sufficiency of Asian refugees (post–Vietnam War, for example) as "models" requiring little financial or other assistance. In the first instance, early Chinese immigrants were reduced to their biological entities, removing them from legal protection. In the second, Southeast Asian refugees were, and still are, subjected to social typings that hinge on visible difference to shape the cultural narrative of the model minority, often to Asian North Americans' detriment.

Even if Chong and Webber do not call attention to race in their drawings, racial constructs such as those exemplified in the aforementioned exhibit "Monsters and Marvels," of ugly Asian tropes and images, continue to influence initial readerly approaches to a graphic narrative by and about an Asian Canadian. Prior encounters with racial types in culture and society galvanize arguments about why race matters in *Dancing After TEN*. In the first fifty pages, Chong's pre-TEN drawings, ripped from a spiral notebook and taped into the graphic narrative (discussed in depth later in relation to my neologism "graphting"), show no distinction between her eyes and skin in relation to those of her boyfriend and peers. All of these characters might be Asian Canadian; all might be white.[13] Later, Webber draws Chong's mother with slightly almond eyes, and after comics avatar Vivian is blind, she is drawn with eyes like sideways carets (< >) that are incontrovertible markers of her Asian identity.[14] They become invisible, or rather not visible, when hidden behind sunglasses. Invisibility advances the assimilative notion of being Asian North American, requiring raced subjects to blend in. To don glasses for sun protection or to shield nonseeing eyes does not erase her eyes as markers of Vivian's Chinese Canadian identity. If a character's nonwhite race is a potential constraint to white readers' identification with her, to remove this impediment casts Vivian as an everywoman, a universal (read white) character. But because her experiences as an Asian Canadian are not universal, to ignore Chong's Asian North American identity is to conveniently circumvent a history of anti-Asian sentiment inferring that Chong immigrated into an imaginary carte blanche. In fact, Canada's Chinese Exclusion Act imposed a Chinese head tax in British Columbia until 1923, it banned most new Chinese immigrants from 1923 to 1947, and the legacies of these discriminatory laws continue to affect Asian North Americans to the present day. A century of trauma leaves generational traces.[15] Expected assimilation occurring throughout this history is an ideological concept attempting to disavow trauma. Vivian, a former Hong Kong citizen, circulates as a marked (racial) body that becomes unremarked within (or as assimilated into) Canada's predominantly white national spaces to affirmative visions of a unified nation—but to Vivian's detriment, to her raced invisibility.

In art, carte blanche refers to the white canvas or white page that invites cartoonists to make their mark. In cultural studies, on the other hand, it references the nation in which colonizers have claimed land, drawn boundaries to their benefit. When the land is deemed empty, pristine, and unmarked, it has rendered the natives, its original residents, as sullied, as those who taint the virgin/pure wilderness and hence require extirpation. A cartoonist's white page is always regarded as already contextualized by publishing requirements—panel- and font-size restrictions, full-color versus black and white—because they are driven by affordability and profit. For instance, color printing is more expensive for both the book industry and the customer than is printing in black and white; paperback copies are cheaper than hard cover. Furthermore, the works of white authors more easily have been adopted than those of their nonwhite counterparts. In the nineteenth century, slave narratives penned or narrated by black authors required the imprimatur of a reputable white writer, which itself did not always guarantee that the narrative went to press. Heretofore unknown autobiographical wor(l)ds required verification by a well-respected white figure that vouched for a black narrative's veracity, even the author's morality, while the white referent was not required to know anything about living as a slave, of escaping plantations, of experiencing precarious "freedoms" of the North about which the narrative spoke. Metaphorically, the white page filled with the hand (writing) and corporeal exploits (and exploitations) of black bodies threatened pride in an abolitionist North and explicitly censured its self-complacency. Such dangerous implications obligated white gatekeepers to pass judgment on the print-worthiness of Black narratives.

The published book is therefore a concept always already bound by requirements, ideologies, and expectations.[16] There exists no truly blank canvas for graphic narratives, especially for artists of color. In her study *Thinking Its Presence: Form, Race, and Subjectivity in Contemporary Asian American*

Poetry, Dorothy Wang "pay[s] serious attention to both the literary and social properties of Asian American writing" because, she argues, "a poem's use of form is inseparable from the larger social, historical, and political contexts that produced the poet's subjectivity" (24). Form, she defines, includes "compositional decisions, structures of language (conscious and unconscious), the shadow of literary precursors" (34). One either can regard Asian North Americans and thus Asian North American poets "as perpetually and constitutively foreign, alien, and threatening" to the nation, argues Wang, or "reward" them with what Mia Tuan calls honorary whiteness, invisible but voiceless, a condition that "grant[s] none of the benefits of white privilege" (Wang 25).

Wang's argument about aesthetics and the racialized poet suggest, on the one hand, that to overemphasize Vivian's Asianness is to alienate her from white readers; on the other, to underemphasize her race is to assimilate her, to endow her with a raceless universality that is not grounded in white privilege and to provide her a subjectivity and agency that elides important, because traumatizing, social, legal, and political histories.[17] Finally, returning to Lee, narratives of the model minority are not armor against failure. Rather, they wound by inflicting increased pressure to uphold the high standards of the myth, continued attempts at its maintenance hiding infirmity while constantly manufacturing it. Paradoxically, depression, anxiety, guilt, regret, or physical frailty are produced by subjects who deem themselves incapable, in their illness, of living up to the myth's high bar.

Clearly, I hesitate to discount Vivian's raced subjectivity, even though one might claim it plays such a faint role for this seemingly assimilated comics avatar who wrestles with blindness, not with racial representation. However, a telling frame near the graphic narrative's conclusion affirms cultural constructions among race, subjectivity, and disability. During one of Vivian's one-woman comic performances, staged years after being afflicted by TEN, Vivian tells a joke that might be easily overlooked (rendered invisible or insignificant) as mere fodder for stand-up comedy routines. Upon closer investigation, however, it is freighted with disturbing racist and ablest meanings attributed to her. She explains to the crowd, "A little kid asks me, 'are your eyes small because you are blind?' Noooo . . ." Vivian croons into the microphone, "it's because I'm Asian" (134). She uses her impairment—blindness—to demonstrate that she is aware that the audience knows that the joke is on her: many Asians lack a double epicanthic fold, making their eyes look smaller than those of non-Asian descent. The latter's possession of the fold is the standard against which Vivian is compared and fails to measure up. She looks / is regarded as different because she is Asian and blind. To attribute the cultural understanding of "difference" to blindness, hence encompassing all blind people whether Asian or not, would no longer be funny in its universality. Blind white subjects might resent this designation. Vivian as the Asian North American object of the punchline is the only way the joke works.

Frederik Byrn Køhlert contends that self-representations on the comics page are an "implicit conversation with an extended history of, for example, misogynist, racist, or ableist visual traditions that artists working in the form must contend with in various ways" (*Serial Selves* 3). As an Asian North American, Vivian's joke contends with, or reduces her to, the biological markers of race at the same time that ignoring race diminishes her as a subject already historically reduced by racism.[18] However, what Vivian knows beyond her audience's ken is that she possesses double vision, understood best through W.E.B. Du Bois's notion of double consciousness: she perceives how her (white) sighted audience regards her and is capable of seeing herself from the viewpoint of an Asian Canadian and a blind woman. Vivian objectifies, through the joke, how others practice an alienation that they cannot themselves discern or do not want to. In discussing common metaphorical constructions between seeing and knowing, Elisabeth El Refaie remarks on the "many feedback loops . . . of visual perception, with the result that our previous experience, knowledge, prejudices, interests, and both conscious and unconscious desires can lead us to see things that are not visible to others" or to not see "the things we do not want to see" (125). Because the quip appears in the last 27 pages of a 161-page graphic narrative, I conjecture that she, Vivian, has possessed this double vision throughout. Despite blindness, Vivian's double vision shames the limited insight of those with actual sight. She reminds us of how she is alienated by both race and disability. She compensates for both by making jokes about herself, inviting white audiences and readers to laugh with her, not at her, even though the joke itself invokes painful histories of racial alienation and unaccepted difference.

I assume readers pay scant attention to decades of racism against Asian North Americans when they read *Dancing After TEN*. They might focus instead on Vivian's gracious acts: she forgives her former boyfriend Seth (in fact, his entire family vacationing with Seth and Vivian), for abandoning her at St. Martin's hospital immediately after she is afflicted with TEN. Their egregious behavior, pardoned by benevolent Vivian, is effortlessly accessible. Readers more easily hold accountable a singular, misbehaving individual (here Seth) for his reprehensible actions than the entirety of a nation, whose discriminatory laws produce generations of (Asian North American) trauma.

Race in *Dancing After TEN* engenders a skirmish between those who look for its resonances (a paranoid reader) and those who do not acknowledge race at all. Validating each stance creates a dispute. If we return to Wang's work to replace "poet" with "comics creator" in the following quote, readers cannot ignore Vivian's race: "For the racialized poet [comics creator], a significant part of her lived and psychic experience is the fact of having moved in the world and been apprehended as a racialized subject" (Wang 36). The cost of ignoring Chong's racial markers in *TEN* is that it diminishes necessary discussions about race. My assumptive reading gives Vivian a raced self-perspective that the graphic narrative's illustrations do not explicitly address. My assertions about race, or my necessary insertions of race, fill a racial gap in *Dancing After TEN* by announcing the gap itself.

In stark contrast to faint traces of race, Chong and Webber never eclipse gender. In fact, in Webber's *Dumb*, comics protagonist Georgia's status us a woman affects how artist Webber curates our reading of her, never allowing her gender to slip from our consciousness. Georgia, for example, develops a public code that will announce daily, depending on her level of pain, her ability to speak or her choice to remain silent. When she wears "lipstick = I am not talking at all. No Lipstick = I will talk a little, if needed" (59). The code, Webber laments, unfortunately associates notions of (silent) women to alluring (lipsticked, self-beautified) women. She questions, "If being a silent woman isn't fraught enough, the addition of lipstick [signaling her complete silence] is disturbing. then what? i'm just decoration? smiling, quiet, made up"? (62).[19] The subsequent page includes a collage of floating lipstick-ed mouths, laughing and smiling; cut-outs of women's eyes looking dreamy or seductive; alphabet letters snipped from magazine print arranged to spell "allure" or "toute femme;" and the drawing of a naked woman's headless body, legs slightly spread over the cut-out letters "OOO" (63). This rash of connections spills onto the subsequent page where more images evoke how "woman" is freighted with social readings and cultural expectations. Georgia eventually rationalizes that if lipstick "really does make it easier to read my lips, so why not? it's not up to me to accomodate [*sic*] potential reactions by avoiding them to begin with . . . if someone else treats me like an object, that's not because i am one" (65). Georgia refuses to hide from potential negative public attitudes related to women who wear lipstick—or not. Writing and drawing out her self-assertion against social inscription are anticipatory gestures of self-representation and self-explanation.

Why not, then, augment race in *Dancing After TEN*? Why not puncture the model minority myth by featuring graphic pathography by and about

Asian Americans whose health fails them, an outcome not controlled by the myth's focus on individual acumen and work ethic?

Graphting: Suturing and Regeneration

Dancing After TEN is an aesthetic regeneration, an innovative product that first limns, then exceeds, through suture and regeneration, the contours of past comics collaborations. Through a term I call "graphting," *Dancing After TEN* constitutes not only a finished work of art but also a new growth, a scion emerging into a powerful, generative, aesthetic entity from two artistic hands. Graphting combines notions of the graft in narrative theory, in medical suture, tissue engineering, and horticultural hybridization. That comics theory references a *graphiateur*, the root of the term embedded in artistic subjectivity, indicates the generative act of drawing itself.[20]

Webber's hand in *Dancing After TEN* is more synergetic than substitutional, the latter describing the many visual, artistic contributions to Pekar's narrative in *American Splendor*. We might begin by regarding Webber's adjustment to Chong's style through medical suture. Suture as a noun is the thread or material used to close a wound; the verb "to suture" is to bind the two edges of a laceration in order to close the divide between them.[21] The process yields a whole from a hole, while traces of this regenerative procedure might be visible as a scar.[22] Regeneration also denotes a process of organic growth, as when skin from a patient's own body or that of another is grafted onto the former to close a tear, repair a burn; their visual amalgamation is the repair. The horticultural graft is also jointure, uniting the sprout or twig of one kind of plant to another. The new growth exhibits qualities of each original in a new entity, a regeneration, while the visible location of their splicing remains. Vivian's surgeon farms flesh from less noticeable areas of Vivian's own body to repair TEN's damages on conspicuous bodily surfaces, practicing medical grafting and tissue engineering (TE).[23] For narrative theorist Gerard Genette, "grafting" posits a hypertext in relation to "an earlier text," a hypotext, "in a manner that is not that of commentary" (5). Through Genette, I contend that Chong's pathography is the earlier text, the original or the hypotext, whose fruition Webber facilitates. Or, we might suggest that Webber's graphic pathography *Dumb* constitutes the original hypotext that inspires Chong to seek her cooperation in *Dancing After TEN*. Their collaboration in the latter becomes the corollary hypertext. Thus, race as embedded in the grapht's base, in its hypotext, cannot serve as a mere footnote in *TEN*.

TEN is more seamless than a tissue graft, yet bears its own scars.[24] The adaptation of one style to another, I contend, can refer to the "dance" of the graphic pathography's title—coordinated artistic efforts between the two artists—and to Vivian's return to an active and fulfilling life after TEN's ravages.[25] Chong and Webber's disability portraiture collaboration simulates that of artist Riva Lehrer, who continuously passes her work, in stages, back to the subjects of her paintings to solicit corrections, additions, more information.[26] In Courtney Lynne Carter's introduction to Lehrer's exhibit, "Consent to Be Seen," she writes, "Through her ethically informed art practice, Lehrer asks how socially devalued bodies are made visible and how portrait-making can intervene in processes of aesthetic and sociocultural revaluation" (quoted in Lehrer n.p.). In this collaborative effort, Lehrer avoids the uneasy territory of depicting what Couser calls "vulnerable subjects," addressed in chapter 3. He is concerned about narratives of disabled subjects who are unable to write/draw themselves, asking those who depict for them if their "representation serves the best interests of vulnerable subjects generally" (*Signifying Bodies* 19). While Chong participates in drawing her own self-image, and commenting on those produced by Webber as Chong's vision wanes, Chong finally wholly relinquishes her representation to Webber when she becomes completely blind. In the spirit of Lehrer, Webber consistently seeks Chong's input during the process of creating the comic. Graphting, then, metaphorically subtends race and healing, wounding and recovery, through artistic endeavors.

Drawing the Lines: Style and Ideology

The artists' intense collaboration on *TEN* over a short ten months also is unusually generative, inviting readers to close the gap between what they see on the page and what can only be inferred. The graphic narrative's aesthetically provocative images toggle between Chong's thready, scratchy illustrations that might express hesitancy, and Webber's strong, black lines, exemplified in her *Dumb*, that might exude confidence.

Drawing's basic element is the line. It connects point A to point B through space. The "process of drawing" lines is "the connection between intimacy, trust, and unlimited discovery," argues Barbara Bernstein (91). Drawn lines that form a dialogue between the nearly unsighted Chong and once briefly silent Webber stitch together *Dancing After TEN*, with Webber finishing what Chong cannot while Chong's abstract work sometimes provides background to Webber's realistic images. At its start, the slight evidence of Webber's substitutional hand might be conceptually understood as subtle dotted lines. Take Vivian's skin grafts, first depicted as pronounced squiggles on her arms and face (*Dancing After TEN* 56). As she heals, they become faint dotted lines (87).

As the narrative progresses, Webber's style presides as dark, bold lines. David Rosand argues that "different modes of drawing represent different modes of knowing" (13). A drawing "mark," he maintains, "is at once created and creating" (7). The texture of a line, thin or thick, sketchy or solid, invests the depicted objects with "associated qualities" (Rosand 8).[27] The "firmer [the] contour," as in what we may assume are Webber's drawings in *Dancing After TEN* that look similar to her work in *Dumb*, the more "confidence as well in the object represented, a faith, as it were, in the continuity of surface, in the existence of the far, unseen side. The very continuity of the line declares that belief" (13). In contrast are the "short, broken strokes" that suggest an object's "boundary" resides in a "liminal zone," akin to a "groping, a skepticism in search of assurance . . . the haptic ambition of the drawing hand" (14). The latter proclamation resonates with what we assume are Chong's scratchy strokes that eventually become nearly nonrepresentational. As Vivian incrementally loses sight of the horizon line, "the far side of the globe" as expressed by Rosand (13), Chong's line embodies that liminality, removed from the surety, boldness, and confidence of Webber's.

Eventually, the book's various drawing styles present visual discord: thready flourishes meet bold strokes; exuberant looping doodles become abstract backgrounds against which minimally sketched human bodies are overlaid. *Dancing After TEN* is an interpolated rapport of styles. As blindness impinges, Chong's hand moves from realistic depiction to abstraction, reflecting her progression from sighted to blind. Or do these lines depict what El Refaie calls a "synesthetic metaphor" (71)? She exemplifies the concept by referencing how the term anger in Ian Williams's graphic pathography *The Bad Doctor* is "translated into jagged lines or spirals around a character's head . . . that translates the experience of heat into particular visual shapes, which itself is based on [a] common conceptual metaphor" (71). Sketches that appear deep in Chong and Webber's pathography—of looping, fluid lines leaning toward adumbration—are, I assume, Chong's abstract backgrounds to Webber's drawings. Do readers also deduce that the heavily outlined, representational figures later in the graphic narrative are in Webber's style in their similarity to drawings from her work *Dumb*?[28] Does Webber eventually manage Vivian's representations on the page while Chong's images function as background (fig. 9)?

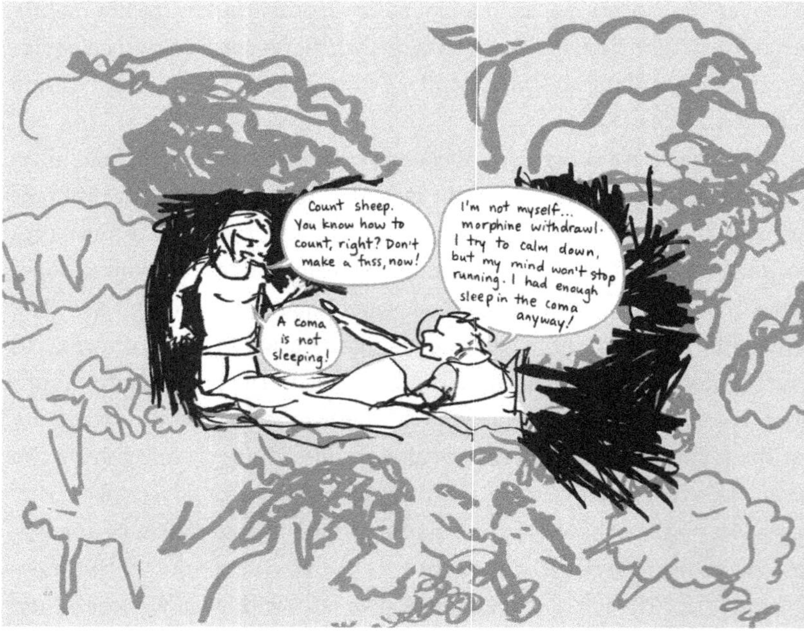
Count sheep. You know how to count, right? Don't make a fuss, now!
I'm not myself... morphine withdrawl. I try to calm down, but my mind won't stop running. I had enough sleep in the coma anyway!
A coma is not sleeping!

Fig. 9 | Is this Chong's self-representation, drawn before her sight begins to disappear, or Webber's assisted interpretation? From Vivian Chong and Georgia Webber, *Dancing After TEN*, 2020, p. 44. Copyright © Vivian Chong and Georgia Webber. Courtesy of Fantagraphics Books (www.fantagraphics.com).

This partnership, where one hand might be indistinguishable from the other, is Chong and Webber's dance, choreo*graphted* through intense communication. Drawing in this graphic narrative is thus artistic graphting, a closure and a regrowth in the stylistic intersection of two hands. Their collective work weaves a new kind of memoir in which the drawing "I" may not always belong to the memoirist herself. Assessed alongside Pekar's *American Splendor*, created by many more than two hands, perhaps both autographics can be considered exceptional.

Finally, Scotch tape is also a suturing material, pasting one thing to another, but in this graphic narrative it uniquely signifies dependency. The adhesive's disappearance from the edges of the same images, reappearing again later in the book, alert us to Vivian's growing independence and healing. Sketches of Vivian's arrival to and initial vacation on St. Martin appear early on in the memoir (13–21). In the original sequence of images, secured by tape to the page, Vivian has just landed on the island with her then-boyfriend Seth, and the couple greets his family. In the image's reprisal—same images, different wording—Vivian has just landed in California to become acquainted with her guide dog. The words in Vivian's speech bubble have changed from "Yeah, we're in St. Martin!" (13) to "This is my decision. My trip. A dog will give me more freedom. This is going to work out" (125). In the latter California sequence, the images bleed seamlessly onto the white page, absent of Scotch tape.[29] The adhesive's disappearance from the edges of images that appear and then reappear alert us to Vivian's growing independence and healing. Furthermore, this slight alteration from the initial sequence marks a positive change in Vivian's stance toward the original scene of trauma. She dispenses with the "support" of an irresponsible boyfriend, metaphorized by the lack of adherents in the California sequence, to depend, instead, on her growing confidence as a nonsighted woman in a world built for the sighted. The smooth incorporation of the final images in *Dancing After TEN* reveal only slight traces of the past—a scarring—in their graphting from the original.

Revisiting the Asian North American Biological Body

I revisit questions posed in this chapter's introduction: Does Asian North American self-representation, when it appears in graphic pathography, change how we assess the model minority? More broadly, would a surge in graphic pathography by and about people of color generally affect our views on race and disease, race and impairment? Vivian certainly delivers a version of the model minority myth: she heals, learns to navigate as unsighted with the help of Catcher, her guide dog, and a cane, and draws and dances once again. She exudes visual embodied authority, health and wellness, in spite of the ravages of TEN. Yet embedded in that achievement are the wounding resonances of race whose contours I have elevated to consciousness. Hence, this chapter addresses two of the book's overarching themes related to graphic pathography as self-care: first, Chong and Webber's images reprimand clinical representations of the pathologized body; second, they undermine cultural and political representations of the Asian North American body, a social justice endeavor.

In this conclusion, I craft a humanist reading of Chong's *Dancing After TEN* that thoughtfully considers the Asian North American biological body and its fragments. In Lee's reading of Asian North American woundedness, he asks us to consider that "a disciplined, healthy body that mirrors the socially and economically productive life she is expected as a model minority reveals the deeply toxic dimensions of such a life" (20–21). Race and biology remain at odds in post-structural theorizing of the cultural and discursive, not biological, construction of bodies, especially those of women and minorities. Yet continued violence and oppression against people of color suggest that the discursive theory of race construction fails for those who depend on validating their own (white) superiority against assumptions of the darker race's inferiority. Rachel Lee argues convincingly that scholars of Asian American studies with interests in self-representation have long desired to pry biology from Western, cultural, and media depictions of Asian North American women which categorize them in stereotypical, usually body-based, types: sexual, hardworking, quiet, disciplined, other-pleasing. Lee, however, notices that in these scholars' claims that race is more than mere biology, they return repeatedly to the material, not discursive, body, to its motions and fragments. Lee's argument relies on the biopolitical body for its potential to reimagine Asian American embodiment as a valuable tool for constructive race thinking.[30] Chong and Webber, too, return to Vivian's biological body as a political move. In one of her most exposed positions, Vivian lies facing us, knees up, feet in stirrups as if for a vaginal exam. Medical staff explain that surgeons will employ "lasers to treat the scars inside your vagina" (50). Chong dares us to gaze at Vivian's vulnerability in this compromised position. At the same time, she resists the fragmentation upheld by sexism, racism, and disability by reasserting her own materiality and bodily integrity. Many of the graphic pathography's illustrations depict Vivian's entire corporeal self on the page, lying on a gurney or in a hospital bed (28, 31, 33, 34, 35, 36, 37, 38, 40, 41, 44, among others). Resilient Vivian discovers that each (drawn) version of herself is stronger than the last as she moves through hospital discharge to living with a helper, from losing a boyfriend to gaining a service dog, the latter highly rated over the boyfriend. Through aesthetic suture with Webber, she pieces together the fragments of herself in this joint venture, learning to dance again.

Echoing the title of James Lee's book, *Pedagogies of Woundedness*, I conclude that focusing on race in Chong's manifestation of embodied disease and impairment is "treacherous," not to Vivian but to accepted assumptions about the intersections of image, race, and pathology within health care's narrow parameters. My race-based approach to *Dancing After TEN* is an adjunct to other pressing issues of race and representation in relation to social justice and equality (here I reference policing, academic arguments about the necessity of creating diverse curricula, voting access, university recruitment, and a myriad of other contemporary race-related issues). Unfortunately, coupled with a dearth of graphic medicine by people of color, the lack assumes that health care and graphic pathography are predominantly white-serving entities. In the following chapter, I turn to work by Ken Dahl (also known as Gabby Schulz) to discuss disease as actants and the devastating effects of whiteness on a white, man character treacherously wounded—rendered deathly ill—by white self-consciousness. What would it mean, Schulz asks, for white subjects to acknowledge race woundedness?

Chapter 6

Vital Viruses

Animating Herpes, Pathologizing Whiteness in Dahl's *Monsters* and Schulz's *Sick*

For artists of graphic pathography, drawing embodiment usefully animates the effects of disease, impairment, or other conditions. Images are emotional and haptic proxies, agential actors. In this chapter, I turn to how germs, viruses, and nonhuman matter become what Jane Bennett calls "actants" collaborating within "agentic assemblages" (*Vibrant Matter* 9, 23).[1] Actants connect—or better yet, cleave—human and nonhuman subjects, where "cleave" denotes both uniting and severing. In her exploration of vital materialism, inanimate matter equally influences and transforms animate beings. Seemingly lifeless elements like minerals or rocks, she alleges, are composed of vital forces acting upon us powerfully and sometimes perniciously, from how minerals of a millennia ago once assisted in creating flying birds and walking humans (11) to the harmful effects of contemporary intoxicating trash accumulating in the wake of humans' excessive materialism (5). Matter's potential to influence is an apt transition from the previous chapter about the social signification of the visible features of race / being Asian and the dissemination of assumed cultural competencies attached to them (i.e., the model minority myth). Human subjects in chapter 5 traverse the cultural thickness of race that depict how ideologies matter. In this chapter, nonhuman substance is a vibrant mediator, alive with conjunctional and transactional possibilities. For Bruno Latour, an actant "is neither an object nor a subject but an 'intervener'" (quoted in Bennett 9). Rather than being acted upon, nonhuman matter arbitrates self-perception, self-consciousness, and interaction with others.

Specifically, in *Monsters* by Ken Dahl (the pen name of Gabby Schulz, who appends the latter name to his publication *Sick*), vital materialism allocates a reading of humans' inhabitation of the herpes virus, defamiliarizing us from an assumed viral occupancy of the human body. Herpes gains an agential viral life in this graphic pathography by initially inhabiting Ken (a white, heterosexual, cisgender man) before forging an existence of its own. While artists use metaphorical monstrosity to self-represent, especially in pathographies, I am not bound to read so figuratively. I uncouple the conventional understanding of metaphor in which the meaning or essence of one familiar concept or object is adopted to describe another, more abstract, idea or notion. I accomplish this through two intellectual moves: I argue that insensate matter in *Monsters* mobilizes to destabilize solidified figurations of the look and feel of illness, which includes how herpes, personified, lives its life independent of host Ken. Subsequently, my argument takes up the physical and social matter of herpes in relation to the materialism of a graphic narrative that can circulate information as it passes from hand to hand. That is, if the highly stigmatized herpes is also extremely ubiquitous, *Monsters* is an unexpected approach to redressing the tabooed status of the herpes simplex virus (HSV). In its dispersion among readers, it spreads essential health information—rather than the virus itself. I begin by discussing the vibrant matter of the nonhuman or the inanimate, as explained by Mel Chen through linguistics. I weave in arguments from Bennett's *Influx and Efflux*, which explain how entities are transformed and transforming in the process of entering and exiting bodies. Ultimately, I turn metaphor inside out by establishing matter's agency: herpes is a metaphorical monster in relation to Ken as well as an individual entity. Their mutual embodiment propels Ken toward a modified understanding of what is monstrous, as elucidated in the chapter's final segment. Through Frederik Byrn Køhlert's discussions about whiteness, white privilege, and illness in Schulz's subsequent graphic pathography *Sick*, I use both graphic works' attention to matter's import as an urgent call to address matters of race.

In Dahl's *Monsters*, the specter of living with (incurable) type I HSV haunts autographical cartoon avatar Ken. He already unknowingly has infected his girlfriend Rory and is terrified of contaminating future sexual partners.

Following an argument with Rory, Ken moves out of their shared apartment and into his father's house, after which he feels intense shame and guilt. In this profound state of emotional angst and self-pity, Ken imagines that he resembles a spiky, slimy glob of HSV goo (54). "Let's face it: nobody wants to fuck a monster . . . and become a monster themselves," he states (55). A panel depicts Ken as a viral ogre devouring Rory—eating akin to infecting her—until she, too, appears as a thorny, salivating beast (55). Feeling doomed to a life of celibacy as an HSV-positive man, Ken's longing glimpses at women bring out a "rabid beast" of sexual abstention and toxic masculinity (71). He is depicted with a canine head, human fingers and feet, dressed in a track suit and tennis shoes. He barks, drools, and growls until a woman passing by with a child gives him an inquisitive "What the fuck?" (72).

Sathyaraj Venkatesan and Chinmay Murali define Ken's imaginative self-representations—a rabid dog, a barbed blob—as expected metaphors: "Dahl in *Monsters* deploys the metaphor of monster to describe the marginalizing nature of illness and forms of othering in its diverse manifestations" ("'I Don't Even Feel Human Anymore'" 79).[2] However, the field of vital materialism provides fertile ground by which to discuss herpes otherwise: the virus as vital actant moves Ken and readers beyond an understanding of HSV as "merely" a figurative beast. Even if the virus is exanimate, it animates transactions within humans that move and influence in two directions: herpes affects humans and, unexpectedly, humans affect herpes. In her *Animacies*, Chen explores the life or aliveness of matter considered insensate or immobile, dead, or what one might call "wrong" (2). In the late 1970s, she explains, linguists approached animacy through discussions about "the grammatical effects of the sentience or liveness of nouns" as opposed to the expectation that only verbs carry action and life. Nouns attain dynamism in this unexpected (turn of) phrase: "the hikers that rocks crush" (2). Rock's animacy and agency over hikers' assumed subjectivity and agency (vitality) disturb accumulated reading assumptions and comprehension. While hikers as active humans are more likely to crush stationary rocks, these inanimate things in the phrasing "the hikers that rocks crush" suddenly inhabit potential vitality, or life, notwithstanding that when large rocks, which we call boulders, fall they can and have crushed hikers. Without context, the awkward phrasing "violates a cross-linguistic preference among speakers. They tend to prefer animate head nouns to accompany subject-extracted relative clauses (the hikers who __ crushed the rock), or inanimate head nouns to accompany object-extracted relative clauses (the rock that the hikers crushed __)" (2). An "animate hierarchy of possible acts" occurs in the sentence "the hikers that rocks crush," according to Chen, interrupting an expected "calculus of animacy" (3).[3] The linguistic disturbance incites productive rereadings of HSV in its commencement of a life of its own.

After Ken is diagnosed with herpes, his formerly mysterious, long-lasting cold sores and painful genital rashes acquire an originary logic. What once was invisible because indeterminate—HSV—materializes as literally and grossly visible to Ken and, he surmises, immediately perceptible to the public. The virus's animation—both as character on the artist's page and in its facility to affect and transform humans like Ken—bestows it with agency. Bayo Akomolafe's argument about "*giving agency*" to the coronavirus in his essay "I, Coronavirus. Mother. Monster. Activist" is useful here. He approaches the virus as a *being* "instead of an annoying glitch in the stock market or a tiny isolatable object [a star light-years away] that lives outside of the kinds of measurements we . . . are making" (emphasis in original). The coronavirus is here among us, this crowned/corona actant inhabiting bodies and lungs similar to the manner in which HSV lodges around Ken's orifices. In its existence as microscopic, however, the coronavirus infects most monumentally, including its effects on education, world economy, and all of global health. The coronavirus moves from the miniscule to the planetary. HSV in *Monsters* moves similarly in Dahl's panels, only to return earthward. Cartoon stars around Ken and Rory's inflamed parts visually symbolize HSV's resultant burning and itching; they mutate first into heavenly constellations (49–50) (fig. 10) before returning earthbound, delineated in medically accurate illustrations (so accurate, in fact, that they may be off-putting to some) in their depiction on lips, labia, breasts, buttocks, inside the mouth, and on a penis (51). Dahl's expansive trajectory moving our perception from the human into the cosmos and back proposes that Ken is a small man in a small world inflicted with insignificant problems, of which HSV is one tiny speck in a world full of more crushing challenges. These overwhelming issues will be magnified in my discussion of *Sick*.

What does it mean for the nonsentient herpes virus to become an anthropomorphized verb, to exist as a being with agency per Akomolafe, to roam from earth to galaxy and back?[4] If I place "herpes" in the same position as "rocks" in Chen's phrase "the rocks that crush hikers" to create the sentence "the people that herpes infects," we are untroubled by the meaning produced. From medical and cultural perspectives, herpes does infect. The linguistic arrangement poses no impediment to comprehension and acceptance that, in passive tense, people are infected by herpes and that, in active tense, herpes can infect people. Herpes is understandably and acceptably

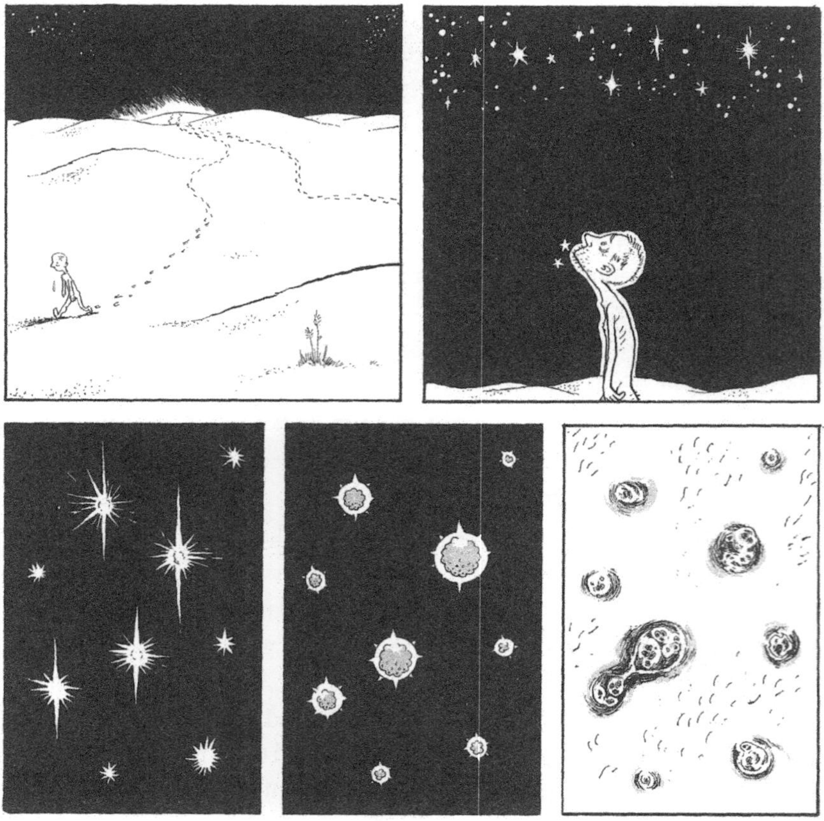

Fig. 10 | Ken's pain *emanata* burgeons into stars, then into the HSV virus. From Ken Dahl *Monsters*, 2009, p. 50.

agential. But if I write, "the infection that peoples herpes," we are stumped, as "people," typically a noun, is now a verb, and herpes is no longer expectedly agential. In Dahl's *Monsters*, what if we insist that HSV can be endowed with personhood? In fact, the virus enjoys an anthropoid social and cultural life. It meets up with friends to chat; it goes to work; it dates (100–106). If animated objects can function as actants, then when Ken peoples herpes, his attitudes vivify the viral blob that he inhabits at the same time that HSV's transparent envelope encompasses/infects Ken.

Herpes emerges as vibrant matter. Once transported by a human carrier, it possesses a life of its own, enticing others into its viable (living) network. That is, the disease's "ecosystem" intervenes in human agency (Bennett, *Vibrant Matter* xviii). The deliberate use of "ecosystem" suggests transference and effect: the loss of one element in such a system affects the life of another. Additionally, an ecosystem is comprised of a biological community (human and nonhuman) in a physical environment (Bennett, *Vibrant Matter* xviii). Ken's ecosystem is inclusive of his self-consciousness about herpes, the physical symptoms of HSV (cold sores, a rash), his sexuality and sexual partners (in potential transmission of the STD through bodily fluids), and the social stigmatization of those "with" the virus. They establish an agential alliance in this animated and animating system. The organizational entity furthermore incorporates clinics, pharmaceutical companies, research labs, and so on in an ever-expanding sphere of significance that, through cross referencing, determines health, defines disease.

This circuit of influence and affect in which nothing or nobody remains unchanged, elaborates Bennett, is "that ubiquitous tendency for outsides to come in, muddy the waters, and exit to partake in new (lively/deathly) waves of encounter" (*Influx and Efflux* x). Terms like transformation, interval, partake, and encounter are evocative of how "the otherwise that entered makes a difference . . . is made different" (x). For Bennett, to engage with poetry, here that by Walt Whitman, is to be open (dilated, a term she borrows from Matt Miller) to "sympathy and understanding," evoking the democratic stance offered by Whitman's work (64). She explains, "He uses poetry to enhance his own and his audience's capacity to detect inchoate flows and signals . . . But the poetry seeks also to alter those currents, to compose them into specifically democratic postures and moods" (61).

Dahl's *Monsters* does not exactly open, dilate, or transform readers. However, graphic pathography taken collectively can expose readers to pulses, vibrations, and sensations expressed in images that, impressed on us, might alter our apathy to others' conditions or diseases. And Ken, who peoples herpes, is affected by and equally alters signals, vibrancy, and the atmosphere of herpes' physical sensations and "public mood," the latter Bennet compares to a "powerful atmospheric current" of anxiety (*Influx and Efflux* 62). In *Monsters*, the *impression* herpes presses upon Ken advances his subsequent *expression*, two terms Bennett finds beneficial to explain the ecological relations between influx and efflux. Impression and expression also exist in comics monstration, defined by Groensteen, as showing through drawing, the marks on the page as descriptive illustration versus the narrator in prose recitation (*Comics and Narration* 37). "Monster" derives from the French term *monstre* meaning to show, to make manifest. Artists accomplish monstration through the hand, "hand" serving as both a verb/action and a noun/style as explained in the introduction. Comics are *mani*festations. Artists' impressions upon the page press upon, or influence, readers whose subsequent affect can positively transform public reception about particular illnesses or impairments—if they so choose. Like Bennett's influx and efflux, graphic pathography's monstration shows where and how it hurts in order to touch, im-press, its readers.[5]

For Jared Gardner, the "hand" or the "line" is itself a circuit whose traces or impressions are revealed in a graphic expression. The artistic line is produced through the appendage's musculature, he argues, but also is governed by the quality of the tools artists use (or can afford), their education, and their environment (socioeconomic class, attitudes, culture) ("Storylines" 67). Gardner quotes comics artist Gary Panter "for [his] sense of the work the line performs in their [cartoonists'] storytelling": "The hand of the line maker is encoded in the line. The heartbeat is visible as are fossils of inhalations and exhalations. . . . The line is a feedback loop" (67). Panter's reference to a line's inhalations and exhalations usefully return us to Bennett's circuitry between influx and efflux. Dahl manifests himself through the line by drawing his cartoon avatar Ken, who is (or both artist and avatar are) influenced *by* the virus, affected *as* the virus, and motivated in relation *to* the virus.[6] Peopled by Ken, herpes is an affective actant that permits Ken to feel, or to be impressed both physically by pain and emotionally through remorse and self-contempt. This "atmosphere" relates to a surrounding ecology loop in which public opinion about STDs influence how STD-infected individuals think about themselves and from which Ken, as a product of monstration, emerges.

Anthropomorphized STDs in Dahl's graphic narrative suggest that those infected are irresponsible, unlovable, and freakish. These judgments press upon Ken as he also experiences the pain of HSV's irrepressible cold sores. In a pre-STD existence, Ken ruminates, he effortlessly navigated in the world, but his HSV-marked (remarkable) body obstructs such a privilege. Consequently, he neither embraces his HSV-infected body nor denies it; rather, Ken peoples herpes.

Unlike Ken, those affected by "monstrous" or stigmatized diseases deliberately distance themselves from their afflictions. In David B.'s *Epileptic*, for example, the artist portrays his brother's seizures as a lizard-like creature with a toothed alligator mouth. The creature relentlessly pursues his brother Jean-Christophe, a looming shadow ready to entwine him unexpectedly in seizure. Jean-Christophe frequently may be enveloped by this behemoth but never becomes one in David B.'s hand. Anorexia for comics avatar Katie, in Katie Green's *Lighter Than My Shadow*, is exacerbated by sexual assault. Her eating disorder manifests in a black, whirling cloud—above, around, sometimes inside her—that she unsuccessfully tries to evade. Anorexia does not become her, but neither does gaining weight; she ruminates to the detriment of her health, an attitude spiraling her consistently into illness. Similarly, protagonist Anna's anorexia in Lesley Fairfield's *Tyranny* is a skeletal scribble anthropomorphizing Anna's inner voice associating extreme slenderness with women's beauty, an equation promoted by media and society.[7] In these examples, the monstrous is a part of and apart from the affected subjects, while Ken fully merges human with monster.

By inhabiting herpes, Ken's bodily surface expands. As a thin character who takes up little space, his growing self-perception as a large herpes blob increases the physical area of receptivity (*Monsters* 54). For Bennett, the more expansive we are in dilation (expanse, here, as surfaces exposed to attitudes and sensations) the better construed to invite atypical (irritating, unusual, different) disruptions to, hopefully, transform us beneficially.

Materiality Matters

Materiality matters to my argument in both Dahl's *Monsters* and (Dahl/) Schulz's *Sick*. I first consider the publications' physical sizes. *Monsters* is small, a perfectly square book at approximately seven by seven inches, as if to suggest the seeming insignificance of harboring herpes, addressed earlier, in a world of more considerable challenges. Conversely, *Sick* is approximately eight and a half inches wide by nearly twelve inches long, its larger material entity encompassing the much more consequential topic of white privilege in relation to racism and oppression. The former fits easily in your hands; the latter is more unwieldy. Each book attests to the simplicity and complexity, respectively, of the sicknesses addressed.

Katalin Orbán's materialist theoretical approach to David Small's *Stitches*, a graphic pathography in which parental indulgences adversely impact a child's health, effectively facilitates a reading of Dahl/Schulz's works. Orbán attends to "both the page [of *Stitches*] as plane and material object and the body as surface and interiority" in her interpretation of how comics avatar David disappears into his imagination as a child (175). He literally dives into the page like Lewis Carroll's Alice into a rabbit hole, she explains. After throat surgery to remove a tumor his parents refused to submit to medical examination over years of its growth, he invites us to tour his damaged orifice. Indeed, he must *show* us the devastating impact of near voicelessness if he cannot verbally *tell* it. His ex*press*ion is monstration. The book becomes "the site of embodied experience," Orbán maintains, "whereby the material object encountered by the reader comes to stand in for the body without reducing that body to metaphor" (180). Such a haptic approach to *Monsters* prohibits Dahl's HSV "monsters" from becoming only—or merely—metaphor. While Ken peoples herpes, the reader does not join him in that inhabitation, as does the reader of *Stitches*, entering David's mouth, traversing with the protagonist between his slippery tongue and giant teeth. In contrast, while Dahl draws us in, he also deliberately keeps us distant. We remain outsiders to Ken's own experience of expulsion, one both self- and culturally imposed. For much of the narrative, Ken is encased in a transparent, spiked bubble, often leaking fluids. His chosen visual self-image represents herpes' social stigma and potential transferability by fluid seepage, a reference to its infection through sexual intimacy. From its capabilities, to its dispersion, to its manifestation in and on the body as sores, and to its longevity—once contracted, it is managed but never fully eliminated—to "have" herpes is to live with the matter corporeally, imaginatively, and eternally. Ken is herpes; herpes is Ken. We view his glum expressions through (underneath and as) the blob's diaphanous outer layer, but we do not enter into his embodiedness (as we did David's mouth in Small's *Stitches*).

Rather, Ken-as-herpes is better explained through affect theory. In Sara Ahmed's *The Cultural Politics of Emotion*, pain and other sensations apprise us of our skin as a receptive surface at the same time that we cannot argue that pain makes us aware of the surface. Skin exists without our conscious awareness of it, except when pricked or aggravated, akin to Drew Leder's absent body, addressed in the introduction, a body more fully acknowledged when we fall ill. That which causes us pain, claims Ahmed, is something from which we move away as it provides "*an impression of a surface*" which is then "*an effect of such intensification of feeling*" (emphasis in original 24). If we stub our toe on a chair leg, Ahmed explains, the phrase "it hurts" permits "it" to reference the toe first, the chair leg next. In the initial instance, "toe" as noun receives the injury; in the second, the chair leg as noun is the injury's source. The latter establishes "bodily relation" to the object that we think created the pain. We then retreat from the chair leg, moving away from the pain, so we imagine, even though we intuitively know it is our brain, not the chair leg, that informs our body, through pain, as a measure of safety. If we were not alerted to painful burns or cuts by quickly retreating from an object "causing" pain, we might inadvertently kill ourselves. In this scenario, we recognize the surface of our skin (the toe) as sensate, argues Ahmed, and that skin does not contain us but rather allows things and others to be "impressed upon" us (Ahmed references Roselyn Rey's *The History of Pain* 25).

Thus impressed and after much resistance, Ken embraces herpes as a moral obligation: he will inform current and future sexual partners that he is,

and forever will be, an HSV carrier. Upon this admission, he receives an unanticipated reply from Hannah, his post-Rory girlfriend, with whom he has not been sexually intimate yet: "I can't believe out of all the things in the world to obsess over, you chose *this!*" (emphasis in original 189). Hannah's surprisingly incredulous response to Ken's dread at informing her, especially given the former 184 pages of self-conscious agonizing over his HSV-positive status, initiates the introduction of a pedagogical stance in the graphic pathography.
Hannah's subsequent speech delivers medical information, incongruous to the narrative's overall tone: "Did you know that like *60%* of American adults have oral herpes?? . . . it turns out that the standard STD test doesn't *even test for herpes!* . . . since so many people have it, and it's incurable, and it's not life-threatening anyway" (emphasis in original 187). Hannah's unexpected mild reaction to Ken's HSV announcement registers her unconditional acceptance of him. Relieved, he unpeoples himself from herpes even though herpes still exists within him as a potential actant. *Monsters*'s concluding image depicts that both vital beings, Ken and HSV, are transformed by their encounter with each other. Leaning on a snow-covered fence, Ken chats with the virus like a friend, the latter grumbling, "I'm just another life form trying to survive in this weird, fucked-up world." Ken affectionately pats the virus replying, "I know, little buddy" (200). They share the last panel of the book in silent appreciation that they forever will be coinhabitants.

Whiteness as Illness and Actant

More considerable illnesses than HSV plague comics avatar Gabby in Schulz's 2019 *Sick*. "Once I got sick," meaningfully announces Gabby on the graphic pathography's first page, defanging the "sickness" of HSV significantly in that *Sick* follows *Monsters* in publication history (n.p.): in such a chronology, was Ken *not* initially "sick" with HSV's sores and rashes before falling ill in this latter publication? In a key critical reading of this graphic pathography, Køhlert argues that Gabby is made ill not by an expected pathogen but by ruminating on his own white race and how that race is implicated in a host of destructive acts ("'Grotesque, Incurable Disease'"). About one-third of the way through *Sick*, Gabby interrogates his status as a white, cisgender heterosexual man, a United States citizen who is enormously privileged despite living in a (noxious) world of virulent corporate greed, latent nuclear destruction, toxic fossil fuels, obstructionist classism, pernicious racism, colonialism, and violence. Reading Dahl's 2009 *Monsters* through vibrant materialism and Bennett's political ecology of influx and efflux lays the foundation for a radical reading of actants, affect, and guilt in Schulz's *Sick*. If *Ann Tenna* by Marchetto offers a corrective to character Marisa's attitudes toward beauty, vanity, and cancer as delineated in Marchetto's *Cancer Vixen*, argued in chapter 2, then *Sick* also provides different, innovative readings of affliction than that presented in the formerly published *Monsters*.

According to Køhlert, Gabby is sickened by the horror of finally and inescapably facing what his (white) race has effected for centuries on brown, black, and native bodies. Gabby agonizes that the virus "from which I once got sick" is, in fact, "people like me . . . [and what they] have done to the world" (*Sick* n.p.). He ticks off a list of atrocities ancient and recent: "eugenics, phrenology, apartheid, gentrification & Zionism . . . nuclear bombs . . . school shootings . . . chemical spills, child-raping priests" (n.p.). Severing the often mutually exclusive connections between race and/as toxins, which Gabby is no longer able to do, is part of what Chen describes as "a decolonial disability theory" ("Unpacking" 29). Chen also reminds us of the presumption of "intoxication, rather than nontoxicity, [which] is to adopt an environmentalist presumption that not all can be known about the more or less universally shared condition of living with 'contaminants'" (28). Gabby is intoxicated by his whiteness, a contamination brought about by capitalism that infects him with negative affects. The condition, while unpleasant, also provides him an opportunity to "converse" with difference, to compare his "thriving" against others' "surviving" (29).

Whiteness (as a race) is typically considered neutral, rendering Gabby's elaborate sickness—illustrated among pages of vomiting, diarrhea, pain, and his inability to get out of bed—generated from acknowledging the tremendous violence attached to a history of the white race an unusually conscientious trope. To be white is to be "at once racially invisible," argues Køhlert, and "at one with the [white] page," hence to be deracinated universally and also in blank, or unshaded contrast to black and brown bodies on the page, that often are depicted through shading (203). An affected Gabby confesses, "I'm extremely grateful for the jackpot of privilege fate granted me when I was born a *white, able, sane, middle-class, cisgendered male* in the 'first world' at the end of the *20th Century*" (emphasis in original n.p.). His privilege is metaphorized as a fat, white baby wearing a crown, dozing in a velvet-lined palanquin. In his sleep, ignorantly oblivious to the wretched landscape of dead trees and half-buried skulls through which he rolls, he clutches a remote control—as if able to change the picture around him on a whim. A driver in a white KKK hood whips ten starving, brown people straining at pulling the cart (n.p.). The "war" he fights is no longer a small, insignificant sickness as

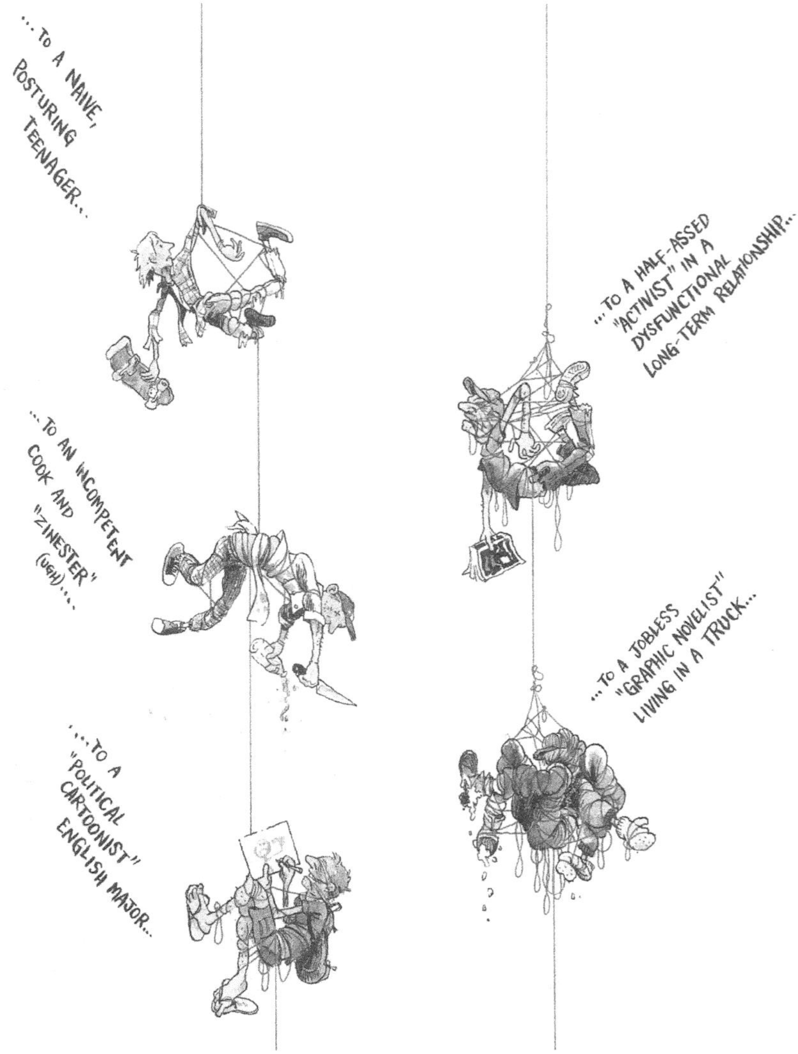

Fig. 11 | Gabby entangled in his ignorance. From Gabby Schultz, *Sick*, 2016, n.p.

in *Monsters* but a grotesque world of demarcations between "the healthy & the sick . . . the strong & the weak, the free & enslaved" that are themselves sick delineations because of the violence, injustice, and suffering these stark distinctions enable (Schulz n.p.).

Through a drawn thread that eventually becomes a sketched net trapping Gabby as he matures (fig. 11), Schulz illustrates how we are entangled in and by vortexes, using Bennett's terms, here of the unacknowledged privileges of (white) race (n.p.). To extricate himself from his line / white lineage is impossible, but he can progress as a human and in the contemporary, damaged world by acknowledging past (mis)deeds, avowing that his "white heritage is toxic," articulates Køhlert (209).[8] Between the publication of *Monsters* and that of *Sick*, between illustrating herpes and delineating living conscientiously in the present by never forgetting the past, Dahl/Schulz radically rescripts answers to "What is illness?" and "Who is ill?"

Gabby Gets Sick While Kimiko Does Cancer

In opening his consciousness to race, the influx and incursion of atrocities committed by white subjects against those with darker skin is of unimaginable horror, so much so that Gabby concludes, "what a fitting punishment to live it" (n.p.). Like herpes, whiteness for Gabby and other white subjects must be lived with. Unlike herpes, whiteness cannot be concealed or even healed by medical treatment. Gabby's compensatory efflux, the best he can do with the tools and circumstances he possesses, is to turn his sickness into art so everybody who reads his work can also be affected and impressed; they can be "sickened" when they acknowledge the (raced) roles they might play when partaking of the world. If Gabby's sickness reminds him that comfort and health might occur at the expense of others, protagonist Kimiko is just such an "other" in *Kimiko Does Cancer: A Graphic Memoir* by Keet Geniza (artist) and Kimiko Tobimatsu (contributor, author). As a Japanese Canadian twenty-five-year-old lesbian with breast cancer, available health care that is informed by Eurocentric and heterosexual ideologies raises challenges and questions for Kimiko that Gabby, a white, heterosexual, cisgender man, need not consider. In fact, ignorance in *Sick* is notably health and wellness for Gabby. Kimiko quickly learns that discussions about egg freezing, paps, sexual health, reproduction, and post-surgery body identity traditionally are pitched to heterosexual cisgender women. As young and queer, currently sexually active with women and undecided about having biological children in the future, she is keenly attuned to the "bad medical advice" she receives, as when her doctor casually remarks upon exiting the exam room, "Only women who sleep with men need paps" (26). Hand on the doorknob, body halfway into the corridor, the busy physician already thinking about her next patient is either unaware or ignorant that Kimiko may want a pap or may desire to ask follow-up questions.[9]

Even if Ken's doctors are equally brusque, the clinic has relied upon decades of research on and about heterosexual health to his advantage as a heterosexual man. Kimiko, however, questions the science of medicine itself. On a waffle-grid page featuring eight talking medical heads, one per panel, each expert offers Kimiko competing information about her cancer's origin, diagnosis, and treatment (*Kimiko Does Cancer* 17). At a breast cancer support group, the three white women who exuberantly greet Kimiko are significantly named Macy, Stacy, and Lacy. Their European rhyming appellations, against which Kimiko's Japanese name grates, reflect the lack of diversity required of such support if it is to be helpful to all women. The so-named triplets are Tobimatsu and Geniza's critique of pink ribbon ideology discussed in chapter 2 in which women in remission are expected to be "survivors, fighters, warriors! We kick cancer's butt! And look good while doing it!" (38) (fig. 12). Those who do not fight similarly become victims of their own passivity, intones the dominant cultural narrative, allowing cancer to win. Going against this cultural grain spells misfortune and failure. For example, in valuing her masculinity, as Kimiko does, she remains inimical to the beliefs upheld by the pink ribbon verbal barrage of these like-named feminine (not necessarily feminist) fighters. In attending the support group, Kimiko desires to learn a variety of coping strategies for those, like her, who affirm their "butchness, dykeness, whatever you want to call it" as they fight cancer (67). However, she quickly grasps that her own way of "looking good" does not accord with that of the heterosexual women in the group, obstructing the necessity for black and brown survivors to connect, and she leaves the meeting halfway through (67).

For Akomolafe, the personified coronavirus remarks that she / mother / the virus makes us human: "We are stowaways in your feelings of grief, in your enactments of joy." White people can more easily stowaway in toxic environments, Kimiko proposes, by listening to (the) others in the room, by toning down white, Eurocentric approaches to living with cancer, to practice gracious influx amid their efflux. If so, can the coronavirus, or cancer, make us more human? Dahl/Schulz's graphic pathographies become vibrant (comics) matter that continue to remind us of our worldly entanglements, our responsibilities, our challenges and privileges, our visibility and invisibility. His incursions into a coalescence of affecting attitudes (influx and efflux) introduce the conclusion's discussion of graphic medicine with and against graphic pathography and the coda's discussion of the visual inscription of race that calls for review.

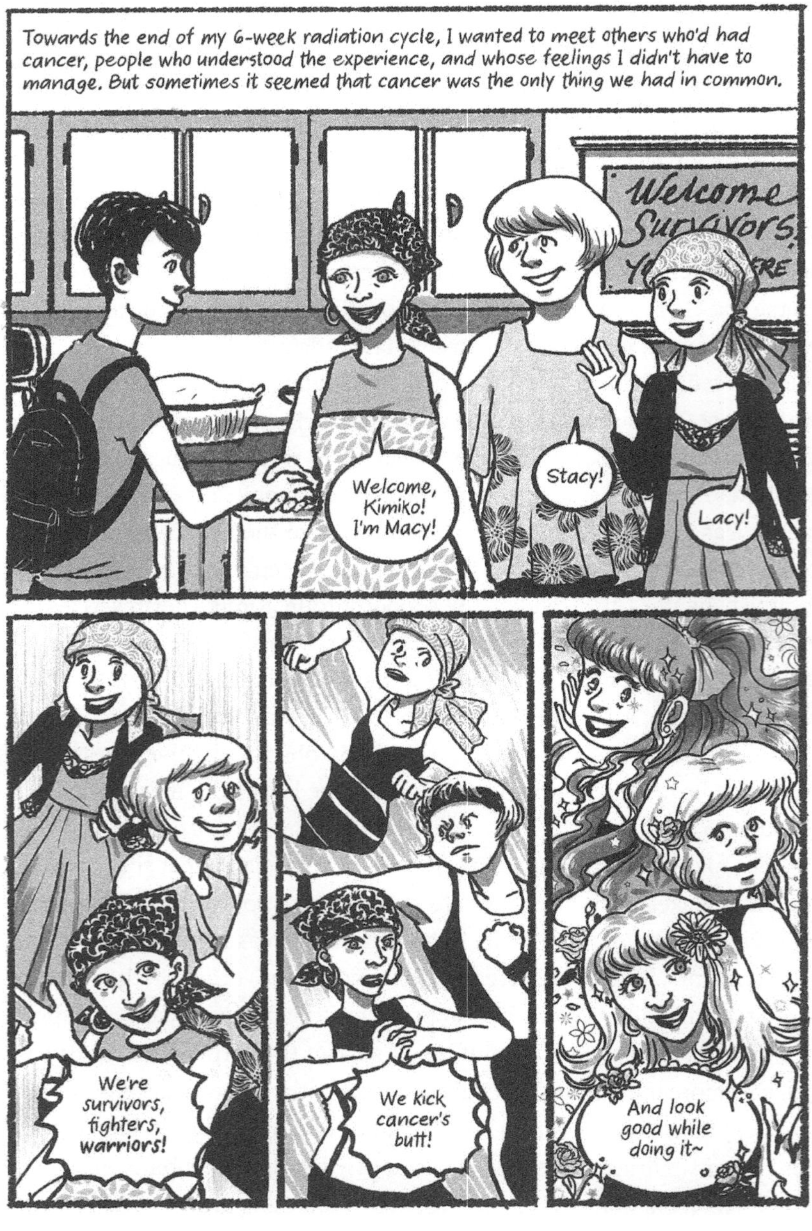
Towards the end of my 6-week radiation cycle, I wanted to meet others who'd had cancer, people who understood the experience, and whose feelings I didn't have to manage. But sometimes it seemed that cancer was the only thing we had in common.
Welcome Survivors
Welcome, Kimiko! I'm Macy!
Stacy!
Lacy!
We're survivors, fighters, warriors!
We kick cancer's butt!
And look good while doing it~

Fig. 12 | The white race/face of cancer and its pink ribbon ideology. From Kimiko Tobimatsu and Keet Geniza, *Kimiko Does Cancer*, 2020, p. 38.

Conclusion

Uncharted: Graphic Medicine by Medical Interns

Graphic pathography critiques a reparative model of medicine that is too narrowly focused on the *soma* at the expense of patients' emotional and psychological reactions to medical care, illness, and impairment. The medium continuously reminds us that well-being derived from experiential (embodied) knowledge and an ethics of care should be mutually constitutive but often are not. Hence, subjects' hand-drawn self-depictions in graphic pathography are resistant drawing; the graphic works reinforce that a sensate subject reacts not only to medical treatment as "merely" a biological body but also to how treatment is delivered by human actors themselves bound up in biopower's influences. In her exploration of portraits, illustrations, and photographs by patients, physicians, and collaborations between them, Ludmilla Jordanova advocates for "medicine *in* art, medicine *as* art, art *in* medical practice, and art *as* medicine (emphasis in original, "Medicine and the Visual Arts" 43). Art, comics art specifically, is the medium for self-advocating.

This study's six chapters argue the following claims. In graphic pathography, cartoonists create an artistic archive of living with illness or impairment. Showing us where it hurts and how through hand-drawn images, artists recover the body through the body. The "hand" is synecdochical. And because "hand" is the comics term for individual, artistic style, it is also metonymical. Graphic pathographies are restorative projects. They reclaim agency lost in the transition from well to unwell and, sometimes, in ongoing, daily living as unwell. They take a position over being positioned. They re-mark—as both commentary and the making of marks—on the literal corporeal positions that confine them to gurneys, examination tables, beds, prosthetic apparatuses, medications, and especially ideologies, drawing against confining historical, institutional and cultural narratives about disease and disability. Falling into, living with, or recovering from disease and disability is so individualized that artists' vast manifestations of conditions of impairment or being unwell create a generative archive replenishing and renewing any static imagining.

As I have argued throughout, graphic pathography educates clinical staff, family care providers, and all those who circulate in the realm of health about manifestations of the so-called diseased or disabled body under social, medical scripts. In what follows, however, I focus on a very different, yet related, type of graphic narrative: I explore graphic medicine by and about medical professionals who engage in dispensing cure to both cooperative and resistant subjects. Their unique perspectives, like those of graphic pathography, also are curated by the institution of medicine.[1] How do the attitudes and opinions of those trained in the system contribute to a fuller picture of health care, I ask. Ian Williams's semiautobiographical graphic narrative *The Bad Doctor*, for example, illustrates his self-doubts, irritations with patients, and perceived failures as a medical practitioner, attitudes affecting his care of them and their attitudes, in turn, about the practice. The relatively new shift from a drawing patient to a cartoon-producing physician makes up the book's final aim, inviting future scholarship and encompassing other actors to show us how it feels to be a provider in the medical system.[2]

Actors trained by the medical system are interpolated within it; their self-representations participate equally in revealing and diminishing its grasp. Reversing the orientation of patients learning from doctors—to medical interns learning from senior physicians, for example—expands graphic medicine by defamiliarizing us from its usual trajectory. It mobilizes another form of resistance by using visual self-manifestations that operate with, not against, those by patients. Esther Szép's definition of comics about the body as "a mediated interaction" is useful here (5). Graphic pathography unites parties through an acknowledgment of mutual vulnerability, according to Szép, between drawing subject and reading recipient. Each acknowledges the other's agential capacities, not only as subjects in Susan Sontag's kingdom of the sick that encompasses all transitions from well to unwell, including recovery, but also as subjects practicing medicine within its institution. The comics *medium* is invested with two objectives: a mode of expressivity transmitting visual self-interpretation, and a bridge between caregivers and their charges. Comics by medical students, practicing physicians, and nurses can enlighten patients to the obstacles and breakthroughs in their own professional trajectory, a deliberate reversal in the flow of affect from patients under medical care. For Sathyaraj Venkatesan and Anu Mary Peter, comics by medical interns in their first year of clinical rotation is an "emerging subgenre of medical narratives" (189). In their "'No Time to Rest, Vent, or Mourn,'" graphic medicine that is created by interns is "a critique of the medical profession" (187) in which trainees experience a "victimization" that demands they hide their "consternation, infirmity . . . [and] inevitable frailties" or "risk . . . punitive retribution" by those in authority (187).[3] How will graphic medicine responsibly attend to my agency, ask both patient and medical student? How does graphic medicine by medical students, interns, and other health care professionals operate to productively critique the profession, as Venkatesan and Peter suggest they can?

Medical students and physicians, like subjects who are ill, also draw against an institutional hierarchy of belittlement by their superiors and training through rigorous rote memorization and repetition whose exercises in bodily exhaustion evacuate instances of emotional connection. Olivia Banner advocates for the benefits of "assigning medical students to observe medical institutions as structures," for themselves and their charges, and encourage them to "imagine structural interventions" (44). Through a mutual recognition between health care provider and patient that their embodiment is mired, albeit differently, within institutionally established conditions of doctoring and being a patient, they draw out new cooperative understanding and new conditions of being on both sides of the medical encounter. Pedagogy should, indeed, work multi-directionally, circulating instructively within an amphitheater of affected and affecting actors. While statistics about how many medical schools adopt reading comics or creating them as integral to the curriculum, and how their success is evaluated, are not available, according to Susan Glazer, comics in medical education are making "inroads" (n.p.). If comics avatars in graphic pathography rematerialize their bodies from disease and redeem their agency from notions of cure to care, comics by clinical staff might repair fraught relationships between patients and themselves, a social justice project of mutual recognition.[4]

Self-Representation as Medical Students' Self-Care

Medical students are often divided from their own bodies in the first two years of their education as they attend lectures, sit exams, and memorize anatomical parts and clinical procedures. During clinical rotations, they practice looking at, examining, and palpating others' bodies whose symptoms and cures often, but not always, correlate to textbook cases.[5] From book knowledge to attending to patients' bodies, students return to the somatic, their own body's submission to a corporally taxing education. While exhausting, the responsibility attached to learning to care also can be awesome, both exhilarating and daunting. In Michael Green's course at the Penn State College of Medicine—"Graphic Storytelling and Medical Narratives"—graphic medicine contributes to medical education, and it is a valuable method of assessing and self-governing one's identity as an emerging doctor. It hones intersections between an individual's experience and a clinical response, contributes Alan Bleakley. Like the patient's bodily manifestation in the drawn line, comics cultivate a "felt response" among medical providers "rather than simply a clinical problem-solving mentality" (17). Bleakley argues that the parsimonious distribution of "sensibility capital" among clinician-educators inspires a pervasive "insensibility" fostered by traditional, hierarchical curricula (19). In thinking through the body, by using their artistic hand to visually express daily challenges or traumatizing moments, students, for example, respond to patient experiences that excite or trouble them. By drawing patients' facial expressions and bodily gestures as well as their own, students productively associate the reciprocity between their words, gestures, and actions in relation to that of their patients. They metaphorically palpate these occasions by slowing down, feeling, and examining them through the pen.[6]

Students explore the effects of medical education on their own performance and the outcome of their own burgeoning clinical practice on those receiving it. In their "Making the Rounds," Craig Klugman, Jennifer Peel, and Diane Beckmann-Mendez report on the success of visual thinking strategies (VTS) for medical students, encouraging deep looking (at art) and deft communication of visual information, essential skills for physicians.[7] Elisabeth El Refaie concludes her study of visual metaphors in graphic pathography by citing their significance in therapeutic and "health communication": "It is now widely acknowledged that the specific metaphors we use to think and talk about a particular disease influence how it is diagnosed and treated by doctors, as well as shaping the attitudes and sometimes even the health outcomes of patients" (188). Central to the curriculum at Peninsula Medical School in England is the application of "life drawing and visual artists" to educate in "close looking in clinical skills" (31, 30). The bulk of *Graphic Medicine Manifesto* posits that students' production of comics—single panels, one-page productions, or zines—are productively pedagogical (Czerwiec, Williams et al.).[8] Williams states that in "these strips, unpolished and unfiltered by commercial editing . . . these artists are producing new knowledge through the intellectual, emotional and manual act of somatic self-expression" ("Portrayal of Illness" 74). Williams bases his assessment on Green's cartooning course, mentioned above, wherein reading comics, which requires attending to relationships forged among words, images, spaces, and time lapses, assists in medical interpretation. The actual practice of medicine also requires a similar piecing together of various presented and invisible data for diagnosis (73).

Perusing Green's website,[9] where he posts selected student comics from his course, 2011 to the present, one quickly finds that many students draw the recurrence of repudiation, humiliation, embarrassment, dismissal, or complete invisibility practiced upon them by their superiors.[10] Numerous cartoons depict attending physicians ignoring a student's appellation on a prominent nametag, preferring to call them by generic terms: "Good job med student" (Holmes, "Good People Great Medicine"); "Speak up intern" (Trey Banbury, "Perspective," 2013), or "C'mon med student. Let's get this over with" (Jeffrey Monk, "A Ghost of an Idea"). In their comics, medical students self-depict being berated by angry supervisors (Andrew Azab, "Feedback") or as victims of monstrous chief residents who literally chew up interns (Banbury). In Shirlene Obuobi's blog "Shirlywhirl, MD," a posting dated 22 February 2022 articulates, "Medicine has a bullying problem. The structure of medical training is highly hierarchical, and trainees are . . . told to be deferential, obedient, restrained. Throughout my training, multiple residents, fellows and attendings have taken advantage of this power dynamic to be demeaning or verbally abusive. The pattern is almost always the same: they are annoyed by a situation, react to it by being abusive toward me, and retroactively declare that their behavior was actually an effort to 'teach' me." Faceless attending faculty lecture from pedestals, depicted as literal soapboxes (as in Shane Lavin, "Whatever Floats Your Boat," 2012). If these pedagogical exercises intentionally humble students to their limited knowledge and skills as emerging physicians, a culturally vaunted position, what effect do they have on both students and future patients? What do students draw otherwise in this medical model? What do they learn from patients that they cannot from often-belittling faculty and supervisors?

Pedagogy based on humiliation or embarrassment deeply and negatively influences students, as they depict in their cartoons. It compels them to doubt their capacity and suitability for the field of medicine and to tamp their enthusiasm about entering a profession of care, especially considering the enormous time and financial commitment to become a certified physician. But many resist in subtle or radical ways. Their resistance, like that of patients in graphic pathography, is a valuable outlet to illustrate their anger and vulnerability in instances of deliberate shaming. They creatively retaliate by demonstrating how connections to individual patients, in concert with knowledge derived from years of study and practice, invigorate their self-confidence and pleasure in doctoring. In "The Honors Game," Luisa De Souza sets her sights on earning an honors distinction in her third year of medical school but feels overlooked for her successes while endlessly chastised for her (expected student) mistakes and missteps. Part and parcel of a medical education is making (correctable) mistakes under the tutelage of guiding supervisors. Her growing uncertainty over a three-day period reporting on a patient under her supervised care is exemplified by the attending and other physicians' bodies growing larger and larger on the page, until the shrinking Louisa reports only to their enormous legs and shoes (fig. 13). She is a diminished figure among the stature of those who make the real decisions in the room. She "earns" a self-defined honors not by impressing her superiors but from the mouth of the patient, who is illustrated at the comics conclusion standing, not lying in bed, after Louisa's proposed treatment protocol proved successful. Intern and patient support each other to stand on their own two feet. The drawing process is thus valuably a self-reflexive process, and if graphic pathography advances patient self-care, graphic medicine offers the same for emergent physicians, as emphasized by Bleakley (62).

Graphic medicine by medical students also provides a necessary and accessible introduction to ambiguity.[11] Medicine often shuns uncertainty and unpredictability. Its confidential stance can assure many an anxious patient. And as with any professional that feels the weight of the imposter syndrome, it builds self-composure. When the overweening pride of supervising faculty psychologically diminishes medical students, however, medicine forgets its foundation in both the unreliability of medicine's positivist science for every body and medical practice as a science *in addition to* a fallible art. For Klugman, Peel, and Beckmann-Mendez "tolerance of ambiguity is associated with physicians being less paternalistic and more open to patients' perspectives" (n.p.). The myriad of decisions students in Michael Green's class make as they sketch out their comics—what to represent and how, how much, from whose perspective will the story be told and why, how will the story unfold—unites the clinical setting, fraught with procedural

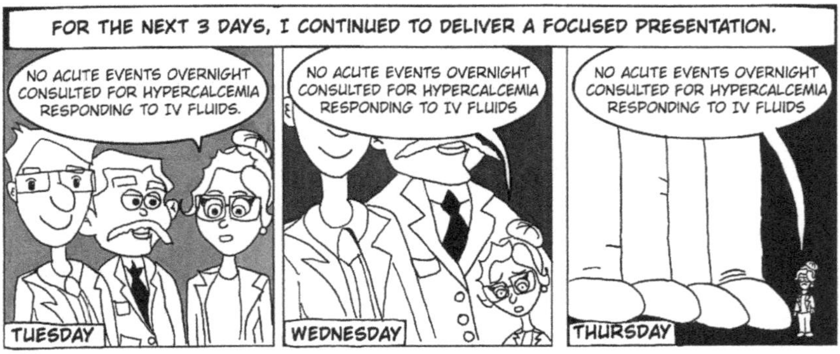
FOR THE NEXT 3 DAYS, I CONTINUED TO DELIVER A FOCUSED PRESENTATION.
NO ACUTE EVENTS OVERNIGHT CONSULTED FOR HYPERCALCEMIA RESPONDING TO IV FLUIDS.
TUESDAY
NO ACUTE EVENTS OVERNIGHT CONSULTED FOR HYPERCALCEMIA RESPONDING TO IV FLUIDS
WEDNESDAY
NO ACUTE EVENTS OVERNIGHT CONSULTED FOR HYPERCALCEMIA RESPONDING TO IV FLUIDS
THURSDAY

Fig. 13 | Luisa shrinks in relation to her attending faculty. From Luisa De Souza, "The Honors Game," 2020. https://sites.psu.edu/graphicnarratives/files/2020/04/Luisa-De-Souza-v2-on-web.pdf. Courtesy of Luisa De Souza.

decisions, and comics creation. Medical students' visual responses to ambiguity, and an acknowledgment of wide swaths of their own ignorance, vitiate their invisibility to each other. The relationship adumbrates a mutual acknowledgment of anxiety (of giving and receiving care), while the symbiosis promotes a mutual recognition of subjectivity and burgeoning agency, first among medical students' peers, then among their patients.

What emerges from these students' comics is an initial adherence to some of clinical medicine's ideologies and hierarchies that might be harmful to care, but which remain convenient traditions based on power differentials to keep students in their place. As many of the comics make clear, students who breach these invisible structures of power—who speak out against sexism or verbal abuse meted out by their superiors, who bravely utter possible counter diagnoses, who spend more time with patients than recommended—discover how patient-centered doctoring requires, then exceeds, book knowledge and rote practice. They individualize their approaches to bedside manner, eventually adopting a style of care all their own.[12] After years of cognitive learning and practical training, they distinguish themselves from "Hey, medical student" to regard themselves and others through compassion and respect. They participate in finding their own agency while also recognizing the agency of their patients. Less a collision of individual and institutional images than pedagogical tools and cooperative imaginings, Jordanova's findings about art in/and/of medicine destabilize orthodox approaches to a distinct separation between art and the practice of medicine. One is neither subordinate nor superior to the other, but they function *in*, *as*, and *with* each other. So, too, might graphic medicine broadly, and graphic pathography specifically within the former's capacious umbrella, encourage how patients and health care providers coordinate effectively in clinical care, as recognizable affective subjects, and with each other, troubling accepted social obstacles to individuality and agency.

If all subjects (here patients and providers) are subjected to conditions of subordination with no conceivable movement beyond circumscription, according to Kathy Dow Magnus (85), the inquiry "'Who are you?' is central to an encounter between two consciousnesses" (Magnus relies on an argument by Adriana Cavarero, 96). "Recognition cannot merely be thought in terms of the subject seeking recognition from the other," she argues, "it must also be understood as the subject approaching and experiencing the other . . . its desire to *bestow recognition* on the other" (emphasis in original 96). Acknowledging the need for an "intrinsic connection with others" expands the task of agential viability from the individual to another who recognizes, or confers upon them, a similarity of constitution (96). Reading is "an ethical act," advances Rita Charon, "joining reader and writer in transformative engagement" ("Introduction" 1). Reading comics about illness creates "empathetic bonds" between artists and readers, say MK Czerwiec and Michelle Huang (they cite Williams, "Hospice Comics" 97).[13] The hospital staff might craft graphic pathography for the patient to read and vice versa, the process vital and affecting for both, Charon would claim. Graphic medicine as a doubled *medium*—as comics and as a bridge—argues its useful reciprocity between physician and medical student, between physician and patient, each colonization by medical education and practice that influence in distinct ways.[14] All groups intentionally stray from a normalizing system when faced with challenges to self-worth, to self- and other respect, to health. What would it mean in health care for each to understand what the other confronts?

In Conclusion and the Afterlives of Graphic Medicine

Chinmay Murali and Sathyaraj Venkatesan vociferously argue that graphic medicine broadly is not merely a "movement" within the health humanities but a necessary "practice" (*Infertility Comics* 19). "Practice" invokes the professional realm of giving care in institutional medicine, they claim, the artistic application to draw toward agency. Susan Merrill Squier pushes us to think even further about potentially transformative contributions of graphic medicine when she relocates the medium out of the medical and health humanities, where it has generally found a good fit, and into "engaged scholarship"

("Uses of Graphic Medicine" 43). She defines the latter as scholarship with "real-world commitment," as in disability studies whose work redefines what we mean by "ability" (43). MK Czerwiec, the self-named Comics Nurse, hopes to read more comics in the future on, for example, "environmental impacts on health . . . about health and social activism . . . [and] access to care" (Kasthuri and Peter 105). Engagement is connection. If health care has developed "from the century of the molecule," argues Atul Gawande, it has landed within "system complexities" (Gawande quoted in Coope 123). I heed approaches through engagement and system complexities when thinking through the implications of our health, wellness, and well-being embedded in North America's developed and materialistic world. Choices driven by convenience and desire result in negative consequences, most often for populations beyond the purview of those privileged with choice.

Graphic medicine can marshal individual agency and disseminate caveats about selfish individualism in our capitalist, materialistic North American world—if we are willing to see them. Jane Bennett's vital materialism, introduced in chapter 6, informs us of beneficial mutual relationship between the inanimate and animate (auguring a posthuman world).[15] Two texts in this study that use each other to test selfish individualism include Marchetto's *Ann Tenna* and *Cancer Vixen*, the former a corrective to "good" women behaving badly. The graphic narratives also engage in environmental justice claims. They dialogue about the adverse, even perverse, connections among beauty, illness, and power in which the fashion industry perpetrates unattainable and unhealthy Western standards of beauty, and about atmospheric toxins causing cancer, which Marisa notes with alarm in *Cancer Vixen* about her work environment in lower Manhattan immediately following 9/11 (32). In other words, if we take up Squier's challenge to produce engaged scholarship, how might scholars' interpretations of graphic pathography resonate beyond the not insignificant patient body on the page, ascertaining connections among agency, social justice, environmentalism, in which universal health care circulates? How might graphic medicine more forcibly attend to an unfortunate historical-cultural entangling of race as disease, taken up in the coda? What social justice interventions will arise in discussing the absence of brown and black subjects in graphic pathography? How might it mobilize beyond so-called mere interventions in attending to individual patients' narratives to fulfill this more capacious goal and venture into new, uncharted territory?

Coda

The Absent Presence of Race: Racial Essentialism and Graphic Pathography

Physician-cartoonist Ian Williams contends that images created for medical pedagogical uses (instructional pamphlets, flyers, signage) remove traces of an individual, neutralizing subjectivity by paring away heads, eyes, expressions so readers can focus on the disease represented ("Comics and the Iconography of Illness" 129). In graphic pathography, subjects respond to neutralization through hand-drawn self-manifestations, as I have demonstrated throughout this book. Olivia Banner affirms that "patients want to be witnessed" (41), to be seen, akin to Tolstoy's dying Ivan, medically looked over, or examined, as a patient by his doctor, but eventually and unfortunately overlooked as a human being. When emotions, reactions, and other human responses to clinical care live on the pages of graphic pathography, they trouble bodily representation determined by what Williams calls "an official iconography that shows how sick people should look ("Comics and the Iconography of Illness" 129). Often underrepresented as sentient beings in clinical care, patients also are overdetermined by race, ethnicity, gender, and economic class. That our nation has cultivated a long history of equating nonwhite races with disease and impairment,[1] graphic pathography curiously lacks a robust collection of visual interventions by people of color, the subject of this coda.

For centuries under overt racism and now under its covert lingering incarnations, people of color have been subjected to unjust violence, have lacked or been denied access to necessary resources, such as healthy and affordable food and housing, sufficient health care, economic parity, stellar education, and respect as human beings. Perpetually fatigued by the "ongoingness of structural inequality and suffering" is what Lauren Berlant calls "slow death" (quoted in Puar 1).[2] It renders them less subjects of disability which, according to Mia Mingus, is a politics of disability for white disabled subjects (Puar 15). Rather, nonwhite subjects of debility face a consistent erosion of the raced body under capitalism. These phenomena chafe against a lack of black and brown cartoonists' self-presentation. Their approaches and inquiries are imperative lest we view cartooning a medium for white people, lest we continue to practice health care geared exclusively toward white people.[3] Encouraging brown, black, and other cartoonists' contributions to graphic pathology is an invitation and a social justice intervention. Rebecca Wanzo, in her *The Content of Our Caricature: African American Comic Art and Political Belonging*, traces black cartoonists over the ages who have employed aesthetics to resist and recast racist caricature and thus injury. We need them now more than ever to redraw images of being injured (ill, impaired) while being black . . . or brown or nonwhite.

If people of color already are pathologized in medicine and society, often debilitated, in relation to whiteness, how will comics about them avoid reinscribing race pathology? Banner, for example, examines "how racism affects medical care" (42) while Stella Bolaki wonders about "the ways in which the categories of race, sexuality, and disability/illness constitute one another" (47–48). This coda is an exploration of this pressing inquiry that, as yet, finds few answers. Furthermore, according to Chris Bell, the field of disability studies is dominated by perspectives of white scholars examining texts filled with white bodies ("Introducing White Disability Studies" 275). Why this steadfast perspective despite Puar's mapping of overwhelming brown and black subjects existing in precarity and debility? Why does the medium of graphic medicine include so few narratives by and about people of color to neutralize this view?[4] Prominent disability scholars like G. Thomas Couser, investigating prose illness narratives, address "the body's form and function (apart from race and gender)"; in his use of parentheses above, identities of race and gender become academic and visual asides (Couser quoted in Avrahami 8). This generates pressing questions about which gatekeepers in the industry or what cultural barriers secure whiteness within graphic pathography and continue to favor graphic pathography by (only) white artists.

In Schulz's *Sick* of chapter 6, I consider how Frederik Byrn Køhlert so cogently argues that Gabby's violent, prolonged illness evolves not from a virus but from acknowledging colonialism, racism, and violence enacted by those of the white race, *his* white race. Embodying whiteness is a disease unto itself. *Sick* illustrates how white, able-bodied, and cisgendered individuals like Gabby possess a much vaster distance from their own skin and their own bodies as cultural, social, historical, and political containers than those of brown and black subjects. Because they can, muses Gabby. Because they have unconsciously accrued benefits from privileges historically denied other races. Their visibility on the page masks a damaging other invisibility. This invisibility is a disease in need of not merely a representational cure but black and brown subjects' own representations as self-care.[5] In graphic pathography's recent meteoric rise against a longer history of slow violence, comics publications by and about raced subjects prevail as key works by which to educate and *impress* a wide range of readers.

In this coda, I first chart a brief history of medical imaging, broadly conceived, as a history of cultural imagining. Medical surveilling techniques, for example, unscientifically manufactured understandings about diseased and disabled white and nonwhite bodies, and a racist form of visual diagnosis practiced at Ellis Island and Angel Island maintained the idea of national health as white health. I then reference graphic pathography by white artists whose work highlights pressing questions about both visualizing and overlooking race as disease.

A History of Imaging, a Culture of Imagining Race and Disease

Medicine has a long visual culture, according to Kirsten Ostherr in *Medical Visions*, ranging from anatomical drawings to the doctor's medical gaze, from microscopes magnifying miniscule elements drawn from the body to those technical visualizing tools, such as X-rays, MRI and CT scans, that penetrate the body scopically; from the use of photography and film to capture so-called deviance in institutionalized patients' visages and gestures to public health campaigns and tv series featuring doctors and nurses (4). She carefully interprets the influences of multimedia images of medicine and medical care on patients and the industry. The very act of imaging bodies, she concludes, projects ideological stances upon them, encouraging images to exceed their original meanings in "extraclinical meanings" (18). We could surmise that attitudes about race are projected into so-called objective research. Lisa Cartwright's *Screening the Body* charts the disturbing history of this visual culture in its political uses as, for instance, an early- twentieth-century "surveillant gaze" (58) and a pseudo-documentary tool in which an "empiricism-visuality conjuncture" could support racist medical views (73).[6] Martin Kemp and Marina Wallace map early "diagnostic" modes of seeing (124), focusing on the advent of photography to create "eugenic records" (134). Such visual evidence supported sterilization campaigns, in one instance. More appalling were eugenicists who found some (often darker) bodies as unfit for life itself, an egregious upshot to how racist ideas come to influence medical care. These studies suggests that researchers often find what they look for, subsequently using those findings to promote subjective, racist ideas.

That science serves politics is a core theme in Sander Gilman's *Picturing Health and Illness*, in which he explores how "illustrated histories of medicine or those histories of medicine that use visual images" become "objects to access cultural fantasies about health, disease and the body" (11). Gilman critiques an erroneous and subjective, hence damaging, use of medical imagery in which images control while illness itself is out of control (32).[7] Immigration histories contributed heavily to manufacturing what Jay Dolmage calls a medicalized "regime of vision" at Ellis Island, a vision that "rhetorically constructed disability and race" (*Disabled upon Arrival* 11, 8).[8] While Dolmage is a scholar of rhetoric, if tweaked, his definition of rhetoric—"the function and circulation of power in language"—could allow visual rhetoric to sustain "the function and circulation of power in [images]" (*Disabled upon Arrival* 9).[9] Under a diagnostic scrutiny he calls an "inspection process" (14), "undesirable bodies"—the "mad," the criminal, the invalid, flawed, and blemished—"were shaded with attributions of disability; and disabled bodies were 'raced' as nonwhite, or as disqualified whites" (17).[10]

Dolmage interrogates immigration, race, and health on the Atlantic side of the United States;[11] Nayan Shah unpacks screening practices of Asian immigrants on the Pacific side, visually patrolling for "the fitness of future citizens" (180), particularly at Angel Island, operational between 1910 and 1940. Like Dolmage, he finds a visual-based examination system scanning these already foreign (alien) bodies for signs of pathology (leprosy, bubonic plague) before extending the exam to internal corporeal systems through inspections of bodily fluids and wastes. The immigration inspection systems managed a huge influx of bodies at both borders and, significantly beyond, as the diagnostic view employed by harbor agents stigmatized those marked as different, understood as deviant. The pathology assumed and then located among immigrants supported convictions of diseased bodies, metaphorically imperiling the nation.[12] So powerful was this prejudiced prognosis in terms of empowering white races and disempowering others, argues Dolmage, that its verbal and visual rhetoric continues to inform medical practices to this day.[13] Banner concludes in her study of structural race in medicine that "Science's delegitimizing of race has not, in other words, brought an end to race's life in medicine, where its continued presence has material effects on how people of color are diagnosed and treated" ("Structural Racism" 25).

We cannot discuss impairment and disability, illness and disease, apart from late-nineteenth- and early-twentieth-century driving ideological constructions equating disease with "alien" immigrants. Cartwright's "empiricism-visuality conjuncture" is a recurring view that continues to affect Asian North Americans over eighty years since the close of Angel Island as harbingers of what former president Trump, referencing the coronavirus, called "the kung flu." In other instances, new remedies were first attempted on nonwhite bodies. In *Silver Wire*, Kriota Willberg, a white cartoonist, illustrates how a cure for fistulas—a postpartum tear between vagina and bladder or rectum from which foul odors emanate and whose leaking materials cause painful skin rashes—came about by practicing on unanesthetized black slave bodies (14). Willberg's drawings mimic the black, flat shapes of paper cuts to illustrate the dark history of this medical procedure, conveying the obscurity of (ab)using black bodies "to give free white women a cure and a life" (16). Harriet Washington's *Medical Apartheid* demonstrates how black subjects, in both sickness and health, provided a foundation for vaccination, surgery, and drug experimentation. Even deceased, black patient Henrietta Lacks's uterine cancer cells maintain a life of their own, as described in Rebecca Skloot's biography of how those cells circulated in labs worldwide in the early 2000s without Lacks's or her family's consent, to benefit cancer research. Despite their vital necessity to white health, black bodies have been ironically tethered to sickness.[14]

In black cartoonist Ebony Flowers's comics vignette "My Lil Sister Lena," from her collection *Hot Comb*, readers are introduced to a nefarious legacy of racist standards of beauty. Lena, an avid baseball player on a young women's team, begins to pluck out her hair, strand by strand, after white teammates tease her about her curls. Two pages of twenty- to twenty-four panels in which a finger is shown plucking out a curly strand of hair emphasizes the painful prick of every pluck as Lena's anxious habit creates a bald patch (fig. 14). She eventually quits therapy and baseball, but she continues to pull out her hair, a strand-by-strand illustration of her enduring life trauma. In *Hot Comb*, Flowers critiques (white standards of beauty) and loves (her black sisters and mothers, in their most capacious definition) by turns.

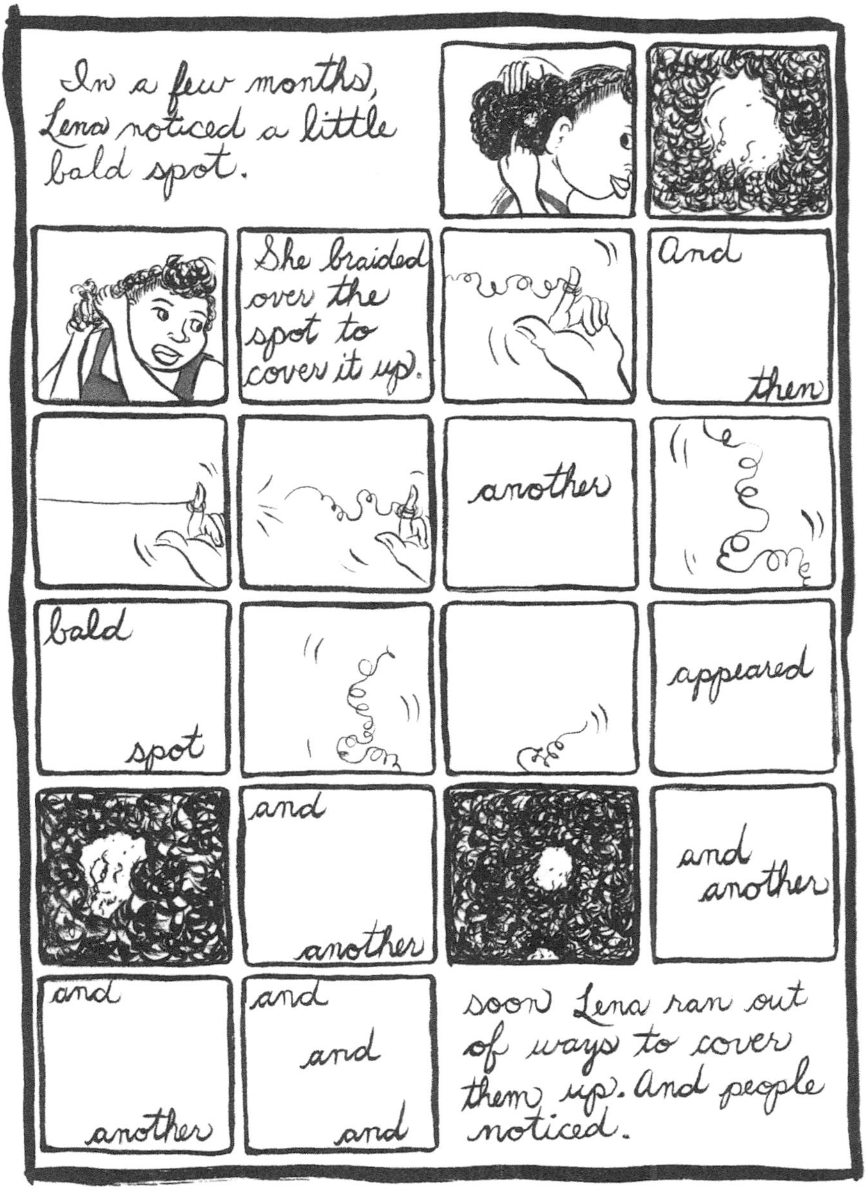
In a few months, Lena noticed a little bald spot.
She braided over the spot to cover it up.
And
then
another
bald
spot
appeared
and
another
and another
and
another
and
and
and
soon Lena ran out of ways to cover them up. And people noticed.

Fig. 14 | Lena plucks out strands of her hair one by one, leaving behind a bald patch. From *Hot Comb*, 2019, p. 102. Copyright © Ebony Flowers. Used with permission from Drawn & Quarterly.

Comics scholarship contributes to the challenge of dismantling racism when it continues to assume white readers and white perspectives, as I briefly allude to here. In her examination of women's autobiographical graphic narratives, for example, Krista Quesenberry finds that "non-human self-representation" in comics offers "an opportunity to strip away many . . . of the visual cues of gender, race, sexuality, and other intersectional identities" (418). Quesenberry argues that the white mother character diagnosed with breast cancer in Jennifer Hayden's *The Story of My Tits* can be depicted "not as a mother or even a woman but as another species [here a doe] in another time and place . . . another sort of being entirely" (419). Based on Quesenberry's argument, should an Asian North American character in graphic pathography be depicted as another species? Who is creating the depiction? To what interpretive goal? Already negatively raced, but simultaneously unremarked in comics, black and brown comics subjects face silencing; their race is all too much "interference or noise," argues Quesenberry, thus deterring (white) comprehension about bodies other than their own (418).

How do readers see and understand themselves in depicted characters? In one of McCloud's oft-referenced theories, he claims that a simplified face, comprised of a circle with two dots for eyes and a slash for a mouth, more easily invites the reader into a character's cartoon world than does a detailed, photorealistic likeness (36). Martha Stoddard Holmes concurs with McCloud that readers see themselves more readily in simplified images of a face. In "Cancer Comics: Narrating Cancer Through Sequential Art," she argues, "We may identify and empathize more freely and fully with cartoon figures than we do with figures and faces that look too much like actual people and thus are clearly not us" (150). If a large portion of graphic pathography is by and about white subjects, elevated by the social institutions that value them, then the "us" presupposes a white icon, and the "clearly not us" assumes not-white iconographic characters. Such a situation requires readers of color to approach texts like a white reader. How does McCloud's reference to readers' self-identification with a simplified cartoon face—often drawn in black ink on white paper—signify across racial experiences?

In "Avatars, Illness, and Authority: Embodied Experience in Breast Cancer Autopathographics," Emily Waples reads the sketchy drawings in *Cancer Made Me A Shallower Person*, by white artist Miriam Engelberg, as visual representations of Miriam's sense of cancer as chaos, wherein "the iconicity of the drawings . . . construct identification with her readership" (177). If that readership is black or Latinx, will their experiences in what has largely been regarded as a racially inequitable medical system be more chaotic and haphazard? Holmes argues that the unfamiliar body or unrecognizable image from which one must "find one's way back to a notion of the self that can be accepted" grates against nonwhite bodies that have been less easily accepted, always unfamiliar and unrecognizable against their white mirror (Holmes quotes from Jane Schultz's essay "(Un)body Double: A Rhapsody on Hairless Identity" 150). Finding oneself strange and foreign during illness is compounded othering for nonwhite subjects, always already foreign and alien against white subjects. If Engleberg's comics avatar is perplexed "about what the [cancerous] body signifies" and that "she no longer knows how to accurately read her own embodiment," as Waples maintains (159), then what does the noncancerous, healthy black body signify; how does this body read itself in a society that daily reads (or more pointedly surveils, polices, and judges) race?

In "Confronting Whiteness: Blankness, Loss, and Visual Disintegration in Graphic Narratives," Xavier Marcó del Pont describes a graphic narrative's unmarked pages as both white and blank, equating this whiteness with loss (254). What is lost when a white subject confronts whiteness; or, in the case of Schulz's *Sick* in chapter 6, what is valuably gained by protagonist Gabby when he confronts his racial whiteness? How can the white characters from Craig Thompson's graphic memoir *Blankets*, or from David Small's graphic memoir *Stitches*, both by white cartoonists, feel lost when they receive multiple representations on the page, visually affirming their worth?[15] The absence of other raced bodies, truly lost from the page, permits society and culture to define them in that absence. How does John Porcellino's vast spaces of whiteness in *The Hospital Suite* impact the white space upon which he is drawn? How does the space of the hospital, filled with white staff, influence him? How would one read and assess that impact? How do we form and reform ourselves with and against imagined and material white spaces?[16] To reckon with race in that space is to uncover a rich range of signification.

Always already othered, black, Latinx, and Asian North American subjects need graphic pathographies by raced artists to un-see how clinical medicine, society, history, media, and politics have already imagined them. If raced bodies are invalid long before they become ill, their depiction on the page by white authors is a disease in need of a representational cure. According to Sara Ahmed, "The more access subjects have to public resources, the more access they may have to the capacity to mobilise narratives of injury within the public domain" (*Cultural Politics of Emotion* 33). When injury "becomes a form of entitlement" (32), she argues, then "the white male subject, for example . . . become[s] an injured party in national discourses . . . as the one who has become 'hurt' by the opening up of the nation to others" (33). Black and brown subjects who are depicted as hurt against always injured whiteness threaten the latter's subjectivity and agency.

Writing against absence affords people of color a capacious opportunity in the medium: there is more artistic and scholarly work to do. This coda is a call to artists of color to draw out their stories of illness and impairment. It is an invitation to scholars to read these manifestations into academic existence.

Notes

Introduction

1. Michael Green and Kimberly Myers define graphic pathographies as "illness narratives in graphic form" ("Graphic Medicine" n.p.). See Anne Hunsaker Hawkins, *Reconstructing Illness*, and Arthur Frank, *Wounded Storyteller*, on the initial use of "pathography"; Martha Stoddard Holmes speaks of "graphic body studies," "a theory and analysis of graphic representations of embodied experiences and social identities" (147). Susan Merrill Squier and Irmela Marei Krüger-Fürhoff use "*PathoGraphics*," also the title of their edited collection, and define "pathography" as "a written, nonfiction narrative of illness" and reference "comics pathographies" ("Introduction" 2, 3).

2. In *Infertility Comics and Graphic Medicine*, Chinmay Murali and Sathyaraj Venkatesan iterate graphic medicine's "critique of biomedicine," accomplished by "recognising the centrality of the patients' voice [in pathographies] which has hitherto been marginalized" (2).

3. G. Thomas Couser advocates that "personal narratives of illness and disability," including "graphic somatography," assist "recovering bodies" in reclaiming "the experience of somatic dysfunction from medical authority" ("Is There a Body in This Text?" 347).

4. This definition is from the *Online Etymology Dictionary*, https://etymonline.com/word/patience, accessed 15 June 2020.

5. Gillian Whitlock coined the term "autographics" in her essay "Autographics."

6. In *Forced to Care: Coercion and Caregiving in America*, Evelyn Nakano Glenn defines "caring for" ("providing for the needs or well-being of another person") and "caring about" ("engag[ing] with both thought and emotion . . . awareness and attentiveness") (186).

7. For social justice issues related to sexual trauma, whose related pathographies I do not investigate in this study, see Courtney Donovan and Ebru Ustundag's "Graphic Narratives, Trauma and Social Justice."

8. In *The Invading Body*, Einat Avrahami speaks of "the body's 'fall' out of categories of normalcy," "a movement from materiality to construction" (9).

9. The antithesis of medical narratives are what Arthur Kleinman calls "illness narratives," advancing how a patient's storied experiences tell a very different account than that of a physician's diagnosis (xii). A medical narrative is a recontextualized diagnosis and prognosis based on physicians' "official narratives like biological science and evidence-based narrative," according to John Launer in *Narrative-Based Primary Care* (2).

10. I thank Becky Karo, emeritus professor of art and art history, University of New Hampshire, for this reminder (email correspondence 19 Oct. 2020).

11. See Lisa Cartwright's *Screening the Body*, where medicine's visual culture stands as a significant obstacle to imaging bodies beyond the public cultures of cinema, for example, that have depended on and iterated mechanisms of medical disciplining.

12. In their *The Graphic Novel*, Jan Baetens and Hugo Frey use "graphiation, "a neologism for 'visual enunciation' or 'graphic expression,' [which] refers to the fact that the hand and the body—as well as the whole personality of an artist—is visible in the way he or she gives a visual representation of a certain object, character, setting, or event" (137).

13. In *Disaster Drawn*, Chute argues that the "power of the hand-drawn image" usefully chafes against media images of war, specifically their "mechanical objectivity," which deviates from the "interpretative" or subjective (112, note 5, 302).

14. From Nate Powell's website: http://www.seemybrotherdance.org/bio/, accessed 15 Sept. 2020.

15. See Barnes's chapter 2 in *The Minority Body*, "Bad-Difference and Mere-Difference" (55–77).

16. Also see Diane Price Herndl's "Disease Versus Disability," terms alternately defined in the medical humanities and disability studies.

17. Barnes, for example, challenges the following accepted definitions of disability in the field: "*Disability is a departure from normal functioning or species of norm*" (emphasis in original, 13) or "*Disability is the lack of a physical ability that most people have*" (emphasis in original, 16). Barnes's *The Minority Body* is a rich resource in which she collapses the distinction between disability and impairment in the social model of disability (25). This model proposes "a moderate social constructionism—a view that says that disability is socially constructed, but which places greater importance on objective features of bodies (rather than how bodies are perceived or treated)," a model that "allows us to say that whether you are disabled is in part determined by what your body is (objectively) like" (38).

18. Ellen Samuels notes that in the United States, other organizations define disability according to the services they offer: Americans with Disabilities Act provides for "reasonable accommodations"; the Social Security Administration is concerned with employment and disability; and Workers Compensation and Veterans Administration calculate loss based on impairment from injury (124). These offices, established at different times and without consultation among them, sometimes work at damaging cross purposes for the impaired subject, declares Samuels (125).

19. In their work in literary disability studies, Jennifer James and Cynthia Wu similarly maintain, through Henri-Jacques Stiker, that those in the Western world prefer to view disabled subjects as correctable, thus avoiding the challenges of "poverty, war, or unsafe industries" that fashion the circumstances out of which many disabilities occur (4).

20. Barnes always carefully distinguishes between "disability" as the form itself and "being disabled" as the effects of ableism (see, for example, 26–27).

21. Barnes notes that she uses Miranda Fricker's definitions of both testimonial injustice and hermeneutical injustice from the latter's study *Epistemic Injustice* (135).

22. Wendell states that the "healthy disabled" are "people whose physical conditions and functional limitations are relatively stable and predictable for the foreseeable future. They may be people who were born with disabilities or people who were disabled by accidents or illnesses later in life, but they regard themselves as healthy, not sick, they do not expect to die any sooner than any other healthy person their age, and they do not need or seek much more medical attention than other healthy people" (19). Wendell does note, however, that "healthy disabled" maintains "a fluctuating and sometimes uncertain membership," as some impairments disappear temporarily then return, allowing for the term "unhealthy disabled" (20).

23. For, according to Zaharijević, if "agency, as a power, cannot lead us out of the field of power" (27)—or, if clinical medicine cannot forge a path outside biopower—is it agency at all? Embodied subjects of agency are a "condition of their access to the world," maintains Zaharijević (22). Kathy Dow Magnus concurs, alleging that while Butler's "subject is *constituted* by social discourse [this] does not mean that the subject is *determined* by social discourse" (emphasis in original 83).

24. Zaharijević claims that the possibility for agency "lies in reproducing or transforming the relations constitutive of our volition" (27). "What we will now," in which "will" is

an enactment of agency, may be "[d]isplacing unwilled effects of the norms (revealing them as unwilled)" (27), an outcome solving Butler's performative "conundrum," as so named by Zaharijević (23).

25. Zaharijević understands agency "as the capacity to perform intentional actions. It assumes that there is an agent who is in possession of capacities and intentions, who is able to self-identify, that is, to validate intentions both as one's own and as the intentions to which one is willing to commit. The holder of this capacity is a self-conscious subject, in possession of the designs of one's will and able to act upon them" (22).

26. See Thomas Patrick Burke's *The Concept of Justice? Is Justice Just?*

27. See *Medical Humanities*, edited by Thomas Cole, Nathan Carlin, and Ronald Carson.

28. See *Health Humanities Reader*, edited by Therese Jones et al., and *Health Humanities*, edited by Paul Crawford et al.

29. In their "Critical Medical Humanities: Embracing Entanglement, Taking Risks," William Viney, Felicity Callard, and Angela Woods list five areas crucial to a more critical medical humanities, of which I mention two: a move beyond the "clinical encounter" and a "closer engagement with critical theory, queer and disability studies, activist politics and other allied fields" (2).

30. El Refaie sketches a rudimentary, two-page history of the origins of graphic pathography, limning much of the territory addressed in Murali and Venkatesan and now, here, by me (54–56).

31. See Joanne Trautmann's *Healing Arts in Dialogue.*

32. Ronald Schleifer, Jerry Vannatta, and Sheila Crow usefully quote Seneca, *De Beneficius* 6.16i n their book *The Chief Concern of Medicine*: "If, therefore, a physician does nothing more than feel my pulse and put me on the list of those who he visits on his rounds, instructing me what to do and what to avoid without any personal feeling, I owe him nothing more than his fee, because he does not seem as a friend but as a client" (Schleifer et al. 137).

33. According to Paul Crawford et al., editors of *Health Humanities*, medical education since the 1900s always has been interdisciplinary: because much good medical work was written in French and German, medical education incorporated language learning; the need to train a diverse population promoted instruction in divergent social realms; and for those operating a private practice, it entailed lessons in economics.

34. Christina Middlebrook wants somebody to ask, "What's it like?" and not to protest or advise as in the following oft-used phrase: "Just think how lucky you are to ______ [fill in the blank]" (Middlebrook quoted in Avrahami 66, 67).

35. Definitions of graphic pathography include the following: Amelia DeFalco posits that "Graphic somatographies are a type of comics that depict experiences of vulnerability caused by illness or impairment, repeatedly drawing attention to the fragility of embodiment and the inevitability of interdependence and care" (224). Emily Waples uses the complementary neologism autopathographics, graphic narratives by and about afflicted artists who use their bodies to reimagine themselves through pen on paper. Anita Wohlmann and Madaline Harrison also use the term autopathographies, which "productively investigat[e]" when "medical narratives often do not match the 'reality' of a disease's progression or the patient's experience of disability" (3).

36. Graphic artists assist in the self-care of other cartoonists, as in Kriota Willberg's *Draw Stronger.*

37. Szép borrows this phrase from Laura Marks in her introduction to *Comics and the Body* (8).

38. *Hogan's Alley* first appeared in full color and on a full page in 1895 in Joseph Pulitzer's *New York World* before appearing in William Randolph Hearst's *New York Journal.*

39. Gardner examines other early cartoons and their connections to illness in "Beyond Metaphor": Winsor McCay's 1903 *Dream of the Rarebit Fiend*, published in the *New York Herald*, depicts addiction to and insomnia from eating too much of the savory cheese-and-bread dish called Welsh rarebit. Gardner subsequently engages with superhero

comics, wherein Batman derives power from trauma, and he discusses women artists who rejected sexualized depictions common in Underground comix and thus contributed to the rise of autobiographical comics by women who depicted their own (sexual) traumas.

40. A number of comics scholars accept delineated eras of the superhero: the Golden Age marking the rise of "firsts," like Superman, Batman, and Wonder Woman; the Silver Age as a post–World War II timeframe launching the well-known Spiderman, initially tepid about connections between power and responsibility; and the Bronze Age, reinvigorating the "silvers" who defied physical aging in the DC and Marvel worlds.

41. For a discussion of sex education comics, see Susan Squier's "Comics in the Health Humanities: A New Approach to Sex and Gender Education."

42. Helen Spandler cautions against "using the term *PathoGraphics* [and thus other terms like graphic pathographies or comic pathographies] . . . [as] it is hard to separate 'patho' from 'pathology,' thus seeming to imply the importance of professional, medical, and pathologizing illness framings" (117).

43. MK Czerwiec, Ian Williams, Susan Merrill Squier, and other authors of *Graphic Medicine Manifesto* are pioneers in graphic pathography in their growing list of talks and academic publications. They continue to champion the medium as comics creators themselves. Both Williams and Czerwiec, for example, teach, discuss, write about, and create their own comics, such as Williams's *The Bad Doctor* and *The Lady Doctor*; Czerwiec is the author of *Taking Turns: Stories from HIV/AIDS Care Unit 371* and edited *Menopause: A Comic Treatment* (an Eisner Award winner). Squier claims the lacunae afforded by graphic narrative (gutters, gaps, distances between images and word and image) map "the erosion of narrative" experienced by those with neurocognitive disability ("Literature and Medicine, Future Tense" 126). The word-image complexity of comics provides the cognitively disabled a medium by which to accurately express their experiences.

44. Social sciences–informed disability studies appearing in the fields of education and disability, especially emerging from Belgium and the Netherlands, are numerous, but they pay little focused attention to nonwhite subjects.

45. For Rosemarie Garland-Thomson in *Staring*, the "normate" is the figure that stands in as—or remains the standard for—the accepted, desired model of humanness: white, cisgender, abled, pleasing to look at, and often male (45).

46. Beyond chapter 5, dedicated to Chong and Webber's *Dancing After TEN*, other references to pathographies by and about people of color receive some limited attention within chapters. I found no suitable place in which to address Teresa Wong's *Dear Scarlet: The Story of My Postpartum Depression* or Whit Taylor's *Up Down Clown*.

Chapter 1

1. These various "selves" are akin to the "serial selves" of Frederik Byrn Køhlert's study of "identity and representation in autobiographical comics," the subtitle of his book.

2. Staring at the atypical has a history. In Rosemarie Garland-Thomson's *Staring*, she delineates a history of "spectacular bodies, those "that are breaches of the common human scale and shape" (161). The idea of the monstrous, a derogatory term to describe the non-normate, has been fascinating to America's cultural, medical, and filmic realms, so much so that staring at that which deviated from the typical became a featured spectatorial event at fairs, circuses, and peep shows, argues Garland-Thomson. Those who were deemed corporeally unusual eventually found their way into medical institutions, removing them from unabashed stares, stigmatizing the person rather than the starer. Graphic pathography allows us to stare at self-described non-normate bodies. But they do so with agendas other than fulfilling reader's curiosities, although see Gesine Wegner's "Reflections on the Boom of Graphic Pathography" for another view.

3. For Sander Gilman, physicians or institutions preferred to control images when illnesses were regarded as "beyond control," manufacturing "aesthetic abstractions" in which "[t]he visible gestures toward the invisible" (32, 37, 36), or the uglier and darker a patient's visage, the further her state from beauty and thus health. While in theory we no longer

assume we can visually ascertain insanity or criminality by gazing at the face, the idea still plays out in everyday social practice, as exemplified in the deaths by police violence of George Floyd, Michael Brown, Trayvon Martin, Eric Garner, and so many more victims of color.

4. For Erving Goffman, traits that "obtrude" from the normate are "an undesired differentness from what we had anticipated" (5).

5. Mitchell and Snyder argue that the "inherent vulnerability and variability of bodies serve literary narratives as a metonym for that which refuses to conform to the mind's desire for order and rationality" (48).

6. Others assume he is emasculated. On the assumption between disability and asexuality, see Mitchell Tepper's "Sexuality and Disability."

7. See Don Kulick and Jens Rydström's *Loneliness and Its Opposite*, in which they discuss how Denmark assists disabled subjects to achieve sexual satisfaction themselves or with partners. Yet in Sweden, a similarly progressive nation, such aid is frowned upon. The authors base their affirmation of Denmark's policies on Martha Nussbaum's "capabilities approach to social justice" which is "a matter of fostering the circumstances that allow individuals to realize a life with human dignity," linking dignity to assisting individuals in what society values (healthy sexual lives) as a matter of social justice (21).

8. See George Lakoff and Mark Johnson's *Metaphors We Live By*, whose title I borrow in my argument.

9. Goffman glosses a history of the word "stigma," a term emerging from the visual cues employed to distinguish a (Greek) slave or criminal body from the rest of the population by cutting or burning them, and from indicators of "bodily signs of holy grace" (embodied by the term "stigmata") (1, 2). He then remarks on current references to stigmata as indications of corporeal irregularity that mark a person as disgraceful.

10. An example from comics that animates how we can read time nonchronologically is Richard McGuire's *Here*. It invites readers to revisit a single place over millennia but not in any chronological order. Moving forward and backward in time, the future, the present, and the past exist simultaneously on the pages. "The end" offers no accepted conclusion to the graphic narrative, the commencement no agreed upon beginning. Had we read from middle "forward," or from the end papers "backward," no different insights would have been gleaned.

11. See Goffman on how society ascribes difference to being not-human, affixes the non-normate with derogatory names, or assigns it "supernatural" qualities that are themselves demeaning despite the positivity bound up in regarding something as "super." Also see Margrit Shildrick's *Embodying the Monster*, on how the vulnerable (disabled, elderly, other) are labeled monstrous.

12. See Paul McIlvenny on page counts for each version, added "sections" in the second publication, and his reading of some of the materials not discussed in my chapter (241). Interestingly, Titan, with DC Comics, also published Frank Miller's 1986 visually and narratively "dark" comic *The Dark Knight Returns*, in which an aging, vengeful, and extremely violent Batman emerges from retirement to rid Gotham City of villains.

13. For Roger Sabin, the move from comics to "'graphic novel' was hype," a public relations gesture that "meant . . . publishers could sell adult comics to a wider public . . . by associating them with novels, and disassociating them from comics" (165).

14. For more on this history, see *From Comic Strips to Graphic Novels*, edited by Daniel Stein and Jan-Noël Thon.

15. In Katalin Orbán's exploration of the tactile materiality of *In the Shadow of No Towers*, a graphic record of Art Spiegelman's reactions to 9/11, the book's size and weight are palpable adjuncts to the Towers themselves. As an usually tall and heavy book, it "weighs on the reader from the start" (172); Michelle Ann Abate charts the rise of board books that invite the very young, who explore their world through their mouths, to "interact with "indestructible" print narratives long before they can read (43). Other graphic narratives with associative haptic covers include the 2020 hard cover copy of First Second's *Dragon Hoops*, by Gene Luen Yang, in bright orange and embossed to replicate the leathery skin of a basketball; and the

2015 hard cover copy of Drawn and Quarterly's *Killing and Dying*, by Adrian Tomine, sheathed in a transparent jacket upon which the title appears in large, white letters.

16. Graphic narrative scholarship cannot but acknowledge the materiality of the page on the reader's posture, or embodied reading. Large, two-page Sunday comics required both hands to hold open the newspaper; meanwhile, children might spread the newspaper out on the floor, lying on the paper to read from top to bottom or vice versa. Materiality makes it presence known physically, aesthetically, and metaphorically. Katie Green's *Lighter Than My Shadow* about anorexia and sexual abuse is, ironically, a fat 508-page tome that weighs on one's reading posture.

17. In "Introducing disABILITY MUNDUS," Patrick Devlieger and his coauthors state that "disability constitutes culture and is not merely influenced by it" (13).

Chapter 2

1. In fact, for Chute, graphic narrative is held up as the most suitable medium for women cartoonists to reveal that which has been concealed about women's sexual trauma (*Graphic Women* 2).

2. In *Screening the Body*, Lisa Cartwright discusses visually "encoded" neurological cases, through subjects once surveilled at the Salpêtriè, "as indicators of a lower developmental or evolutionary state" (51).

3. As I learned from reading the sole footnote in Antonio Ferraro's essay "The Price of an Ending," Marchetto, now divorced, currently publishes under the name Marisa Acocella, but because this graphic narrative was published under her married name, I continue to refer to the author as Marchetto throughout, as does Ferraro (note 1, 162).

4. Marchetto plays with visual metaphor: SuperAnn's elevated speech consists of words created from astral-looking alphabetical letters. Her shoes are equally hierarchical and uplifting. With heels as tall as ladders, she walks in the air, even on the air, tutoring Ann to rise above, but for the longest time, SuperAnn's entreaties are to little avail.

5. An initial selection arguing the rise of such phenomena includes Thomas Laqueur's *Making Sex* (1992); Ludmilla Jordanova's *Sexual Visions* (1993); and Londa Schiebinger's *Nature's Body* (2004).

6. Gilman charts a history of medicine and visual culture from the fifteenth century to the 1990s. His concluding chapter addresses visual representations of AIDS appearing on public health posters at the height of the AIDS crisis.

7. See Gilman et al., *The Face of Madness*; and his *Seeing the Insane*.

8. Avrahami maintains that prose "[i]llness narrative enact[s] a movement from materiality to construction that occurs when one's body suddenly grows out of step with one's psyche . . . the body's 'fall' out of categories of normalcy instigates the writers' and readers' reevaluation of the relationship between the discursive and the real" (9).

9. My use of the term "afterlives" is informed by Ari Larissa Heinrich's *The Afterlife of Images*.

10. For Eve Kosofsky Sedgwick in *Touching Feeling*, "an affect theory is, among other things, a mode of selective scanning and amplification" (135), thus allowing gay and lesbian Americans to select or choose the subjects to which they might direct their negativity. Additionally for Sedgwick, "affects can be, and are, attached to things, people, ideas, sensations, relations, activities, ambitions, institutions, and any number of other things, including other affects" (19).

11. In *Ugly Feelings*, Ngai explores what she views as "lower passions" in relation to other "canonical emotions," in which irritation animates Ngai's work about the emotion of anger, while envy provides fertile literary ground over the "higher passion" of jealousy (11).

12. From a cognitive and behavioral view, emotions can be "caught" by which we synchronize or mimic them, argue the authors of *Emotional Contagion*, Elaine Hatfield, John Cacioppo, and Richard Rapson.

13. "Of particular interest is facial expression's activation of a mimetic impulse in response to the facial expression of observers, tending then to elicit the same affect in them. It is very

difficult not to respond to a spontaneous smile with a spontaneous smile of one's own, and one's own smile provides sufficient feedback to our own bodies to activate the physiological and neurological aspects of joy" (Anna Gibbs, 191).

14. Berlant exemplifies this defeat in her reading of Charles Johnson's short story "Exchange Value" in which two poor African American protagonists discover that having (stealing) money to purchase coveted objects of desire will not "buy" them the belonging for which they long. Acquiring desired goods does not provide the requisite agency to enjoy them, rendering the optimism itself cruel.

15. Eli Clare argues, "Certainly ending environmental destruction will prevent some body-mind conditions. But by bluntly leveraging ableism, the ads [by the Sierra Club on the relationship between coal and asthma] conflate justice with the eradication of disability. The price disabled and chronically ill people pay for this argument is high. It reduces our experiences of breathing, of living with conditions deemed birth defects, of having cancer, of learning in many different ways to proofs of injustice" (56). What about "the damage caused by ableism," he asks (56). Or "How do we witness, name, and resist the injustices that reshape and damage all kinds of body-minds [as they are entangled in subjectivity] . . . while not equating disability with injustice?" (56).

Chapter 3

1. Physician Barron Lerner claims that narratives by patients about their ills and the care they receive show "dissatisfaction with a patriarchal and authoritarian medical system" (quoted in Judy Segal's "Breast Cancer Narratives as Public Rhetoric" 6). While autopathographies, as Segal calls narratives written by ill subjects (6), abound in relation to cancer, especially breast cancer, no single such graphic pathography exists in which a subject records her aging process. What does this suggest about what topics make for "good" or popular reading?

2. See Ai-jen Poo's *The Age of Dignity*.

3. In Barbara Frey Waxman's *To Live in the Center of the Moment*, she argues that these texts and her readings of them "can transform our fear of aging and our wariness of elders" (2). Kathleen Woodward asserts, "The problem here is in part precisely that of *representing aging primarily in terms of the body*. What of the psyche?" (emphasis in original, Woodward quoted in Waxman 8). Chast's graphic narrative focuses on the "limits age imposes" on the body and the mind (Waxman 8), while Farmer's depicts bodily decline in the midst of bolstering life memories/psyche through objects: dolls, family collections, and other material stuff to be discussed in this chapter.

4. More examples include Paco Roca's fictional *Wrinkles* about a character with Alzheimer's recently arrived to assisted living; Lucy Knisley's *Displacement: A Travelogue* visually records her grandmother's growing dementia through a journal Knisley keeps when on a cruise with her grandparents; and Rebecca Roher's *Bird in a Cage* illustrates early-onset dementia, brought about by a head injury, suffered by the author's grandmother.

5. Kerrie Kemperman provided this insight (personal email correspondence 30 Sept. 2021).

6. While I puzzled over the title *Special Exits*, I thank an anonymous reviewer of my manuscript for alerting me to the work's original cover featuring character Lars, seated in front of an open door, watching Charon row by, as if inviting Lars into death.

7. Can Chast harm or wrong her parents in the vein of G. Thomas Couser's definitions in *Recovering Bodies*: harming suggests "adversely affecting someone's *interests*, while *wronging* involves violating someone's *rights*" (emphasis in original, Couser quotes Beauchamp and Childress, 76).

8. Kemperman's critiques of my approach to memoir are well taken: "The criticism of self-indulgence seems to be leveled at every memoir writer. The ethics of writing memoir, a narrative in which the writer is intimately involved, means the writer *cannot* leave themselves out and still call it a memoir. Memoir writers do need to interrogate their own character on the page as much as (or more than!) others represented in the book. The writer can't speak for others, but can depict them, their words and behaviors, and the writer can reflect on their

own histories and interpretations of shared events (personal email correspondence 30 Sept. 2021).

9. Henry Jenkins calls her line "jittery," a "nervous, unsteady hand" that makes the characters "jiggle before our eyes" (n.p.).

10. One also might argue that Chast captures the energy of New York City in her animated style. This, especially in Chast's *Going into Town*, contrasts to Julie Wertz's own comics love letter to New York City: *Tenements, Towers and Trash*. While Wertz's drawings are filled with detail, so much so that one could gaze for hours at New York's architecture, its bicycles, signs, and storefronts, it is a city devoid of people. The sidewalks of the Big Apple's past and present are oddly empty of humans.

11. In his reading of Brian Fies's *Mom's Cancer*, Antonio Ferraro claims that the "cruelty" of medical caregivers has the "capacity to impact the entire family . . . [and] how the consequences of illness and medical treatment often transcend the individual" ("The Many Fictions of Illness" 244).

12. According to Chadwick Roberts, *Tits and Clits* contained "explicit content . . . largely meant not to titillate [as it might suggest from its title] but to bring a woman's point of view to discussions of sex [especially women's sexual pleasure] during the apex of the sexual revolution" (18).

13. It is available here: http://www.ep.tc/eve/index.html, under the pseudonyms Chin Lyvely and Joyce Sutton. Information about Farmer is available at the Graphic Medicine Website: http://www.graphicmedicine.org/Laura-farmer-sex-politics-and-aging-parents/, accessed 18 Jan. 2019. By 30 September 2021, the material was no longer available at the site.

14. For Chute, this practice makes visible once obscured upheaval; suffering effects of the Holocaust, of atomic bombs on Hiroshima and Nagasaki, or the ravages of war on civilians in places like Gaza and Palestine forces us to confront any idea of an "objective" or "realistic" historical report (Chute, *Disaster Drawn* 199). Trauma propels Chute's scholarly work. Formerly silenced and invisible traumas of sexually abused women cannot be unseen once they have been vividly illustrated in graphic narratives. In speaking of Debbie Dreschler's semi-autobiographical *Daddy's Girl*, Jane Tolmie argues similarly that the given images in graphic narratives about the sexual abuse of children by their fathers does not leave "the mind free to refuse to imagine in ways that the image does not" (xiv).

15. Roz illustrates Elizabeth's decline into inept housekeeping (15); Elizabeth's choice to drive herself home, sight impaired, after cataract surgery (23); her intention to save money on a new heater (for their fifty-eight-degree apartment in winter) by filing down a prong on a three-pronged plug on a "space heater from when you were a little baby" (26); and other practices Chast presents as the ridiculous and dangerous antics of the aged. Dominant two-page spreads, which almost always contain a punchline, toe this line as well: "A Rare Sex Talk" or "Dirty Checkers" and "Sheer Lunacy" (25, 33, 47).

16. I agree with Hannah Miodrag on the affect of Burns's style in his *Black Hole*: "It seems to be these even, tessellating lines that create in Burns's drawings a sense of something living, faintly palpitating, and thus an attendant impression of a kind of squirming movement in these neat barbs" (201).

17. Chast is attracted to the idiosyncratic, as photographs of peculiar six-knobbed red and green standpipes or a scarlet and gold hydrant named "Trixxxi" appear in her subsequent graphic narrative *Going into Town* (63).

18. For Nancy Pedri, a photograph inserted into a graphic narrative is "a hand-selected artefact, one that gains meaning within the universe in which it was transposed" ("Cartooning Ex-posing Photography" 253). While Pedri finds that cartoons "carry more weight for what concerns the truthful rendition of selves" (this argument appears in her investigation of Marisa Acocella Marchetto's *Cancer Vixen*) (260), I find a nostalgic emotional tenor in Chast's photo gallery of stuff that resists the irritation present in most of Chast's cartoons.

19. For more on the scholarship of things, see the following: Daniel Miller's *Stuff*; Sherry Turkle's edited collection *Evocative Objects*; a special issue of *Critical Inquiry* dedicated to the theory of "things."

20. In her 1999 *Love's Labor*, Eva Feder Kittay assesses the status of "dependency work" (ix), which Glenn, in 2014, calls simply "care." I find it fascinating that the two scholars argue from what we might call opposite sides of the caregiving equation, Kittay investigating the person dependent on care, Glenn the person giving the care. What has animated this linguistic change (dependency work versus care), thus political change?

21. Glenn also advocates that "high-quality care" be "equally distributed and not dependent on economic or social status" and "the responsibility and actual work of caring are relatively equitably shared so that the burden of care does not fall disproportionately, as it does now, on disadvantaged groups—women, racialized minorities, and immigrants" (189).

22. Goto's concern for queer and biracial people of color is rooted in her appreciation of the lands on which she resides as a former "emigrant from Japan who gratefully lives on the Unceded Musqueam, Skwxwú7mesh, and Tsleil-Waututh territories" (from inside the jacket flap of *Shadow Life*, the 2021 First Second hardcover edition).

Chapter 4

1. I acknowledge Yi-Fu Tuan's elaboration between space and place, the latter an arena imbued with social, political, historical, or personal meaning.

2. See Courtney Donovan's "Graphic Pathogeographies" in which she defines "health geography" as "not only how the physical environment of health facilities has bearing on the subjective experience of individuals who seek care but also how this experience can have broader implications in how health and health care is experienced at the scale of the body" (274, 275). She investigates how place affects the protagonists and family members of David B.'s *Epileptic* and David Small's *Stitches*, both graphic pathographies.

3. In *Graphic Women*, Chute claims that graphic narrative "pushes on conceptions of the unrepresentable that have become commonplace in the wake of deconstruction. . . . Graphic narrative asserts the value of presence, however complex and contingent" (2). Subsequently in her 2016 *Disaster Drawn*, she argues that the hand-drawn style of comics and its "unique spatial grammar of gutters, grids and panels" contribute to documentary comics' aesthetic and political significance for witnessing history (4). For Kate Polak, "The formal qualities of graphic narratives—including the gutter, the stating of point of view, and the textual-imagistic hybridity—make them uniquely suited to questions relating to how we negotiate representations of extremity" (2). Artist Nye Wright contends that "comics are the *perfect medium* for exploring the *universal* and yet still *taboo* subject of the *human journey* through *medicine* (emphasis in original, quoted in MK Czerwiec et al., eds., *Graphic Medicine Manifesto* 172).

4. The popularity of TV soaps and series whose narratives play out in hospital settings, from *General Hospital* to *St. Elsewhere*, from *Grey's Anatomy* to *ER*, dramatize events along a trajectory from the waiting room or ambulance to the surgical theater. Much happens, they regularly depict, in the seemingly static space and condition of waiting.

5. Charon articulates five narrative features of medicine, one being that of temporality, or how the practice "is suffused with attention to life's temporal horizons," however, she does not provide a definition of "horizons" (*Narrative Medicine* 39).

6. For theories about comics in relation to linguistics, see Neil Cohn's *The Visual Language of Comics: Introduction to the Structure and Cognition of Sequential Images*; and Frank Bramlett's edited collection *Linguistics and the Study of Comics*. On visual rhetoric, see Nicholas Mirzoeff's *The Right to Look: A Counter History of Visuality*; and Laurie Gries's *Still Life with Rhetoric: A New Materialist Approach for Visual Rhetorics*.

7. The exception is an examination of buildings-as-property in Chris Ware's *Building Stories*, featuring a brick apartment complex filled with colorful characters.

8. Richard McGuire's nearly wordless graphic narrative *Here*, a biography of a fictional house—or more specifically its *living* room and the uses to which it is put—from prehistoric past to the imagined future, is an excellent example of what Gaston Bachelard calls the poetics of space. The house itself as subject and object conjures aesthetic and emotional memories and projections of its own intimate house-ness. I also acknowledge Ware's fascination

with physically bisecting buildings as if they were bodies, wherein he metaphorically cuts them from sternum to pelvis or peels back their skin/brick walls. Lefebvre suggests that if we remove the brick and concrete façades of a building, or remove their "glorified screens," we reveal "streams of energy which run in and out of it by every imaginable route: water, gas, electricity, telephone lines, radio and television signals, and so on" (93). The immobility of the building as physical bricks and mortar is revealed to be "an active body" that requires "massive energy supplies" (93).

9. Pierre Bourdieu's concept of habitus is useful for unpacking the interrelations among actors or characters in the spaces of comics panels. The habitus is an embodiment of the capital that subjects bring into their environments. Bourdieu's capital includes material wealth one accrues and the knowledge and social practices inherited from family, learned in school, church, and/or other influential institutions or relationships and bequeathed from institutions of higher education and employment. Embodied practices in spaces are those produced by habitus, ways of acting or thinking accumulated over time and class, and by the kinds of capital (cultural, economic, educational) that people bring with them into spaces (Bourdieu and Wacquant 101). In concert, Joe Painter asserts that "[i]ndividuals bring to the field both the embodied dispositions of the habitus and their stock of accumulated capitals" (245).

10. The protraction of space encourages prolonged reading time and lengthened diegetic time as Paula and Tamar walk the wing's extended length. While the empty halls suggest an environment of silence and slow, deliberate motion, the panels also possess an embedded momentum. Readers are stopped at the double doors with Paula and Tamar but, like the characters themselves, are compelled forward by the diegesis, advancing to the subsequent page in a Western left-to-right reading progression.

11. Will Eisner discusses how to use perspective to promote a reader's feelings of insecurity or safety in *Comics and Sequential Art*.

12. A view of the monster from below, states Eisner, "evokes a sense of threat," while "there is little threat or involvement" if the viewer watches the monster from above (92).

13. Amid the consistency of panel variety, only Ware's inclusion of paper cut-outs in *Jimmy Corrigan* indicate where and how we might find difference in the graphic narrative. Ware urges readers to snip out and assemble the three-dimensional models from a two-dimensional piece of paper. He invites an unflattening of space against the consistently one-dimensional Jimmy.

14. In their essay "Graphic Whiteness and the Lessons of Chris Ware's *Jimmy Corrigan*," Juda Bennett and Cassandra Jackson argue that not only is Amy, the black subject, given control over Jimmy, an unstable white character, but she also is given the last word—or the last image—in the paperback edition, permitting her to be "imagined as separate and independent from Jimmy" (n.p.).

15. Jimmy's grandfather was abandoned by his own father at Chicago's 1869 World's Fair, a child in his nightshirt left alone among a community of strangers. The Corrigan family is plagued by legacies of desertion.

16. The ER waiting room is one of the graphic narrative's smallest spaces, apart from incidents occurring in the expectedly reduced spheres of a car's passenger seat or an airplane's economy-class seat. Interestingly, though, while both modes of auto and plane move Jimmy's body, he himself remains immobile, psychologically, throughout, his comics soundtrack a singular, unwavering note.

17. Ware's addition of a postscript about Amy, in the paperback edition, begs related questions: Is it a snapshot of Amy's past, or it is her life in the future, after James Corrigan's death? If the reader can choose, then her selected orientation motivates one meaning over another. As such, is Amy freed from the linear trajectory of black women's roles in "caring for" white people or is she tethered to the reader's assumptions about what black women should or can do well—nursing? What does this postscript extension (or is it an augmentation, a progression?) say about Amy's race?

18. See the following for more on how whiteness operates in *Jimmy Corrigan*: Bennett and Jackson's "Graphic Whiteness"; Xavier Marcó del Pont's "Confronting the Whiteness"; Paul

Williams's "'A Purely American Tale'"; James Ziegler's "A Secret History of Miscegenation"; Joanna Davis-McElligatt's "Confronting the Intersections of Race, Immigration, and Representation in Chris Ware's Comics."

19. The depiction of peaches, scattered throughout *Jimmy Corrigan*, references Jimmy's grandfather, who was once gifted a box of peaches.

20. In contrast, they point to Paula Knight's graphic memoir *The Facts of Life* that "allows the author to arraign the ideology of pronatalism as an oppressive force that mediates her lived experience of infertility" (*Infertility Comics and Graphic Narrative* 11).

21. In *No Future*, Lee Edelman avers that queerness resists heterosexual reproductive futurism in which the child, who embodies the future, privileges heteronormativity (2).

22. Is medicine "a science and an art?" asks Kathryn Montgomery (*How Doctors Think* 30). She finds the clinical aspect of a doctor's profession more akin to social science than medical science, as doctors rely on "the relatively subjective skills of physical diagnosis" (30). See specifically her chapter "The Misdescription of Medicine" (29–41).

Chapter 5

1. Ann Jurecic writes about how to approach this new form—the autobiography of illness—in her *Illness as Narrative*.

2. For a rare example, see Lan Dong's essay "The Model Minority Between Medical School and Nintendo," where she draws out the "nuances and complexity of the model minority myth" (84).

3. He also goes by the published name Christopher Bell.

4. In Zoe Thorogood's fictional graphic narrative *The Impending Blindness of Billie Scott*, young artist Billie is given only a few months, before she completely loses her sight, to execute ten original art pieces to fulfill the obligations of a received award. In an aesthetic representation of impending blindness, Thorogood employs an increasing number of black blobs on the comics pages, slowly obscuring Billie's view and our view of the page.

5. I note Gertrude Stein's 1933 *Autobiography of Alice B. Toklas*, which names Toklas as someone who is not the author of her so-named autobiography.

6. Bredehoft concludes that in choosing an artist like Robert Crumb for his distinctive style, Pekar undermines the usual separation between the author who writes the narrative and the artist who creates accompanying images (102). In *American Splendor*, he explains, the chosen illustrators are "full-fledged authorial partners, situated in an 'authorial' position every bit as powerful and important as Pekar's own" and "we must conclude that the work [or each vignette authored by Pekar and illustrated by his chosen artist] has two authors" (103, 104). That is, artistic style is authorial in and of itself.

7. Information about his parents, Samuel and Dora Pekar, is from *The Encyclopedia of Cleveland History* https://case.edu/ech/articles/p/pekar-harvey, accessed 12 Mar. 2022.

8. For an introduction to the partnership between Webber and Chong, as they explain it, see https://www.youtube.com/watch?v=g3R8ka4n4Mo.

9. See Monica Chiu and Jeanette Roan's essay "Asian American Graphic Narrative."

10. Ironically, another argument suggests that a deliberate separation of people of color from white people might reduce raced bodies to a collective, as set forth by Cassandra Jackson in her exploration of black subjects in photography's art world. They are never individualized, she claims, "but instead . . . always the representative of the collected other," an "emblematic body" ("Visualizing Slavery" 33).

11. Until we learn that TEN is an acronym for toxic epidermal necrolysis syndrome, we might assume that "TEN" is a time (as in ten o'clock) after which somebody goes dancing.

12. For Ty, "hieroglyphs" are signs of race in the shape of the eyes, color of the hair or skin, contours of the nose and body. Hortense Spillers speaks of the "hieroglyphics" of race, the scars slaves and freed blacks bear from beatings, brandings, bullets, and other traumas to the flesh (67).

13. Webber's ethnic identity also is unmarked, but the use of black (round) dots to symbolize her eyes in her memoir *Dumb* strongly channels whiteness. That she does not shade her

comics avatar's skin also delineates a drawn, or perhaps undrawn, whiteness. Vivian's (non) racial depiction is the universal whiteness with which white readers identify.

14. A colleague who read an early draft of this chapter suggested that the editorial carets also can signify that something is missing. Is it race? Is it sight?

15. For more on generational trauma and traveling trauma, see Christina Sharpe's *In the Wake: On Blackness and Being*; Resmaa Menakem's *My Grandmother's Hands* (he argues that even European bodies passed on trauma to other European bodies, later instilling it in African slaves); and Jeffrey Alexander et al., eds., *Cultural Trauma and Collective Identity*, among others.

16. In *The Novel and the Police*, D. A. Miller argues that to draw against or not to draw at all both result in the same empowerment of the institution (of arresting crime in the novel *Oliver Twist* from which he makes his argument). The attacks launched against institutions of the police, of capitalism, of poverty, for example, are the repeated actions by which they remain in existence and on which Charles Dickens bases his novels. The medium of comics, so auspicious for depicting anew women's traumas (Chute, *Graphic Women*) and health and mental health (Pedri and Velentzas) now joins this exceedingly occupied "blank" page.

17. According to Wang, terms such as "transnational," "global," or "diasporic," chosen by academic institutions to rename departments or courses, demonstrate a decisive "mov[e] away from having to deal with issues of US racial politics—and racism," a shift away from a more conscious emphasis on (domestic) Asian American studies (28). See specifically her chapter 8 (272–305).

18. In a historical amalgamation of Asians as masses or hordes stealing jobs or overtaking the nation, as argued by Colleen Lye in *America's Asia*, their individuality recesses. In a historical focus on singular body parts—almond-shaped eyes, so-called yellow skin—the parts take precedence over the whole.

19. Jay Dolmage and Dale Jacobs, who discuss Webber's codes and collage of images, state that "lipstick itself is a symbol of female objectification" (24).

20. Graphiation is "directed to the graphic trace and gesture, and ultimately the artist's subjectivity," states Kai Mikkonen, who uses terms from French comics critic Philippe Marion (112).

21. I acknowledge suture theory in film studies and literary studies, but it is only obliquely related to how I use graphting as suture in this chapter.

22. In *Silver Wire*, a comics history of suturing techniques, Kriota Willberg connects medical suturing to "domestic sewing," traditionally performed by women: "For a millennia, surgeons have been closing up the body with threads, wires, knots, buttons, pins, and beads. There were the same materials used for sewing textiles in the home" (1).

23. TE is an emerging technology that relies on a patient's own tissue by which to grow needed organs (livers, skin, corneas) for "autologous transfers," reports Melinda Cooper (104). TE eliminates consternation over organ expiration dates on transfers from other bodies or the wounding frictions of an artificial steel prosthetic. TE relies on a body's ability to grow itself, from cells onward, in an unobstructed process of self-regeneration.

24. Vivian's healing is a regenerative process that ironically depends on unhinging herself from dependence not just on sight but also on intimate partners, family, Chinese cultural practices, and even illustration, which is her beloved profession. Vivian's morphogenesis occurs against the grain of what we might view as typical adjuncts to the healing process.

25. Webber calls their collaboration a dance in the Youtube video "*Dancing After TEN* graphic memoir by Vivian Chong and Georgia Webber" at https://www.youtube.com/watch?v=g3R8ka4n4Mo.

26. I thank one of the manuscript's anonymous readers for introducing me to Lehrer's "Consent to be Seen," an exhibit of her collaborative work in Haverford College's Magill Library, October 2016 to January 2017, curated by Courtney Carter and Kristin Lindgren.

27. Rosand's conclusion that the quality of a drawn line might express confidence or exhibit liminality also rests on assumptions bedeviled by ideology: in our western society, or among European artists, why does a solid line represent confidence? Can it also represent arrogance, a veil for feeling inadequate? Might thousands of short, fractured strokes— attesting to hours

of pen work—such as those of Julie Doucet's *My New York Diary*, attest to artistic audacity and dedication, both indications of confidence? We are socialized into thinking and believing, even when reading a line, that bold is strong hence good, and that sketchy is weak hence bad. Yet in the art world itself, we find a host of contradictions at play between chosen line and its content: Picasso's fractured (broken) faces depicting three angles at once are outlined in bold brush strokes; the seemingly stringent separation in Mark Rothko's color-block paintings, upon closer examination, betray fades between, say, bright red and brilliant orange; Art Spiegelman's clear-line figures of Jewish mice and German cats against shaggy backgrounds in *Maus I* and *II* depict the bravery of the former during the Holocaust and the reprehensible actions of the latter—despite the ragged lines. The lines question which is more exceptional: survival amid unimaginable fear or the audacity to commit genocide against an entire ethnic group?

28. In a discussion of notions of sculpture and stasis in Mike Mignola's graphic work, Scott Bukatman associates "seething energies" to Jack Kirby's fluid lines (149) and the "*absence* of movement" (emphasis in original 152) to a favoring of "mass" and "*implied* time" (163, 172).

29. Proof that the images torn from a notebook are Chong's include references in a video about the artists' collaboration (See https://www.youtube.com/watch?v=g3R8ka4n4Mo, accessed 29 Jan. 2021), where Kathleen Rea, the graphic pathography's editor, holds a sheaf of papers torn from a notebook, explaining that she and Chong were discussing the possible dance-theater piece when, says Rea, she "brought me 100 pages of an unfinished graphic novel" that told her story. The pages in her arms contain those pulled from a spiral-bound notebook.

30. Alexander G. Weheliye argues that fragments of the body can be politicized: "Poetic assemblages" of bio fragments in spaces like Guantanamo Bay, prisons, internment camps, reservations are "racializing assemblage[s]" (13). Weheliye succinctly states, "If the body represents legal personhood qua self-possession, then the flesh designates those dimensions of human life cleaved by the working together of depravation and deprivation. In order for this cruel ruse to succeed, however, subjects must be transformed into flesh before being granted the illusion of possessing a body" (39).

Chapter 6

1. Bennett is influenced by Bruno Latour, who describes an actant as "something that acts or to which activity is granted by others," and it need not be human (quoted in Bennett, *Vibrant Matter* 9). She turns to Giles Deleuze and Felix Guattari for insights into assemblages, which she describes as "ad hoc groupings of diverse elements, of vibrant materials of all sorts. Assemblages are living, throbbing confederations that are able to function despite the persistent presence of energies that confound them from within" (*Vibrant Matter* 23–24).

2. In her *Teratologies*, Jackie Stacey mobilizes metaphorical language as a balm: if we do not utter the term "cancer," but rather metaphorize it, "perhaps cancer does not have to be confronted" (63). In the Merriam-Webster dictionary, she finds the definition of "teras": "an organism (as a fetus) that is grossly abnormal in structure due to genetic or developmental causes," or a monster (63). She argues, "Metaphors rush to the rescue of the subject whose terror is otherwise uncontainable. Metaphors provide the necessary balm for the psychic pain of the unbearable knowledge. Metaphors enable us to detour around undesirable subjects" (63). For Susan Sontag, however, metaphors of illness are unfortunate negative tropes that obscure disease while casting shame on its bearers.

3. See Chen's racialization of lead in *Animacies*' chapter 5, "Lead's Racial Matters."

4. "[W]ithout a visa. Or a brain," Akomolafe writes of the coronavirus, "the virus [as a lifeform] jumped across bodies, slinked its sensuously shaped protein exterior across handshakes, slipped into nostrils and cracks on the skin surfaces, got spat out and sneezed out on doorknobs . . . flew in first class from terminals in Europe and Asia and the Americas . . . melted through our affection and hugs . . . and settled in our lungs."

5. Hillary Chute attests that "comics is a way for [Alison] Bechdel to touch the subjects on whom her work focuses" ("Comics Form and Narrating Lives" 113).

6. In "Comic-Grotesque Metamorphoses: Boundaries Between Illness and Health in Ken Dahl's *Monsters*," Christina Maria Koch notes "the disturbed unity of the subject" in which Ken and "the monster" are sometimes one, other times separate entities (153).

7. For cartoon avatar Élodie, of Élodie Durant's autopathography *Parenthesis*, the book's title announces how a cancerous tumor causes epileptic seizures whose visual incarnation as parentheses on the page also imagistically separates and adjoins the time before and after a "spell" (30).

8. The image resonates with one in Green's *Binky Brown Meets the Holy Virgin Mary* of a trussed-up Binky, hands tied behind his back, entangled in his religious proclivities and distressed by his OCD. He hangs from shackles that bloody his ankles over a piece of paper on which he is drawing panels with his mouth (n.p.).

9. Remarking similarly about her employer, she wonders, "Why are law firms still so white?" as she sits in a nearly empty subway car during her commute home, the dark panels of this page reflecting Kimiko's unhappiness (34).

Conclusion

1. I acknowledge a variety of health care providers whose practice falls beyond that of the insensitive doctor, curt nurse, or other actors that patients have confronted in graphic medicine. Anne Whitehead in "The Medical Humanities" reminds us that the medical humanities emerged in the postwar 1960s when clinicians themselves "questioned traditional ways of doing things," and were especially suspect of the "technologisation" of medicine and "market pressures" on care, looking to the humanities for alternative views (Whitehead quotes Ronald Carson, 109).

2. Susan Squier and Ryan Marks state that "comics created by physicians and psychiatric nurses, such as Ian Williams's *Bad Doctor* and Darryl Cunningham's *Psychiatric Tales*, are puncturing the myth of Doctor Kildare [a character from a 1930s and 1940s television series] and uncovering the personal vulnerability of health care workers, as well as their struggles with institutional medicine" (150). Also see Susan Glazer on Williams's influence and other graphic pathography in her article "Graphic Medicine."

3. Venkatesan and Peter discuss the many changes to education in health care, for example "the commercialization and privatization of healthcare" in which interns are "increasingly regarded as resources of hospitals rather than students whose chief purpose is to learn to be skillful physicians themselves. Increasingly exploited as the source of revenue rather than serving as apprentices, interns risk depression and in some cases, even suicide" (188). Furthermore, interns' "brutal work culture" seems antithetical to the "academic disposition of medical education itself" (188).

4. For a sampling of essays that address the value of the humanities (narrative medicine, graphic pathography) in clinical education, often with a focus on cultural competence and social justice, see the following: Anita Wohlmann and Madaline Harrison's "To Be Continued: Serial Narration, Chronic Disease, and Disability"; Arno Kumagai and Monica Lypson's "Beyond Cultural Competence"; Delese Wear et al., "Cultural Competency 2.0"; and Delese Wear's "The Medical Humanities: Toward a Renewed Praxis."

5. In *The Lady Doctor*, Ian Williams usefully employs a twelve-panel waffle grid, each frame depicting a patient's quirky face or a close-up of a body part with an injury, visually reflecting general internist Lois Pritchard's sense of an unending queue of patients (see 69, 109, 175). Jay Baruch notes, "To become an excellent doctor, one must take care of patients, an endless train of them" (514).

6. For Abraham Verghese, "the body is the text, a text that is changing and must be frequently inspected, *palpated*, percussed, and auscultated" (emphasis added, 2749).

7. VTS is based on three broad questions: "What do you see? What do you see that makes you think that? What more do you see?" (Craig Klugman et al., "Making the Rounds" n.p.). The teacher repeats what the student sees, moving to the next student to ask the same

question, build upon, or refute the first view, and so on around the class, strengthening listening and collaborative skills and honing observational muscle, necessary for students' future clinical rounds (Klugman et al., n.p.).

8. In Kimberly Myers's course for medical students, carefully reading body language, gestures, and expressions deployed by protagonist Marisa in Marchetto's *Cancer Vixen* and the character's health care providers educates them in being attentive to what patients do not say and to check constantly the cues they may be passing along through their visage, posture, and tone of voice (93–97). Green, who also assigns *Cancer Vixen* in his Penn State College of Medicine course for fourth-year medical students, finds that Marisa's dramatic reactions help "students experience at a visceral level the feeling of being on the receiving end of" bad news, exacerbated by its transmission, from a physician, in "routine conversation" (75).

9. See https://sites.psu.edu/graphicnarratives/.

10. Also see Harmon Fong's digital "Call" about a resident in family medicine: http://www.medthics.com/07.html.

11. For Klugman, Peel, and Beckmann-Mendez, visual thinking strategies (VTS) cultivate "an increased tolerance for ambiguity or uncertainty," endemic to the health care profession (n.p.). Also see Alan Bleakley on "homeostasis" in arts versus its status in medicine ("Medical Humanities" 210; and his "seven steps of ambiguity" 211–15).

12. Verghese states, "For the clinician, the bedside is hallowed ground, the place where fellow human beings allow us the privilege of looking at, touching, and listening to their bodies. Our skills and discernment must be worthy of such trust" (2751).

13. Not everybody agrees that the introduction of the humanities into medicine helps shape more humane practitioners, as outlined in the "Introduction" to *Health Humanities Reader*, edited by Therese Jones et al.

14. Glazer quotes Green's acknowledgment, "'There's not a ton of data yet' on whether comics improve diagnostic skills or foster empathy among medical students. Similarly, there's not much research on whether comics are a more effective way of informing patients about their medical conditions than straight prose or other forms of media" (n.p.). Also see Bleakley on "measuring the immeasurable" ("Medical Humanities" 207). He quotes Rita Charon, who wonders if "One can and ought . . . to try to measure . . . that aspect of learning which is meant as an antidote to the reductiveness of the curriculum" (208). Other sources: Jakob Ousager and Helle Johannessen's "Humanities in Undergraduate Medical Education"; Louise Younie's "Art in Medical Education." Finally, see Lara K. Ronan and MK Czerwiec's bibliography to their "A Novel Graphic Medicine Curriculum for Resident Physicians." They conclude, "While this study was not able to determine whether the curriculum had an impact on burnout symptoms, it does suggest that despite those symptoms of burnout, a graphic medicine approach is an acceptable mechanism to convey meaningful content to busy, stressed and burned-out residents. . . . The readings evoked empathy and understanding of the value of effective physician/patient and/or care-giver communication" (577).

15. See also Mel Chen's *Animacies: Biopolitics, Racial Mattering, and Queer Affect* on mediations of dead matter living culturally destructive lives. I am referencing her discussion of (dead) lead and the life it leads as a dangerous, environmental actant on, predominantly, children of color.

Coda

1. See Jennifer James and Cynthia Wu's "Editor's Introduction: Race, Ethnicity, Disability, and Literature."

2. Slow death, according to Berlant, is "a condition of being worn out by the activity of reproducing life" (quoted in Puar, *The Right to Maim* 12).

3. In "Structural Racism and Practices of Reading in the Medical Humanities," Olivia Banner argues that Anatole Broyard's *Intoxicated by My Illness* (1992), used extensively in the field of narrative medicine, obstructs readers' ability to ascertain his race, to contextualize it in a field in which uneven care between blacks and whites contributes to prolonging illness and invites closer scrutiny of race in medical context (34).

4. One response might blame comics industry's gatekeepers. Bart Beaty and Benjamin Woo in their *The Greatest Comic Book of All Time* explore what cultural barriers secure whiteness within graphic pathography and generate graphic pathography by white artists? Beaty and Woo argue that "great" is less about a work's inherent literary value than the "shared context" assessing it, assessors often white and cisgender (4).

5. Another reason for this invitation is outlined by self-described Mia Mingus who yearns for "access intimacy . . . that elusive, hard to describe feeling when someone else 'gets' your access needs" ("Access Intimacy: The Missing Link," mentioned in Puar's *The Right to Maim* as such: "disability justice activist Mia Mingus, who identifies as a 'queer, physically disabled Korean woman transracial and transnational adoptee'" [15]).

6. Such views included that epilepsy in women and black men was innate, requiring surgery (67), whereas white men might potentially "self-correct" (66); that dystonia musculorum deformans is "genetically recessive among Jews" (73).

7. Far from realistic or mimetic representations of ill bodies in the real world, Gilman explores the "self-contained visual language or iconography concerning health and illness that exist in specific traditions of visual representation and as objects to access cultural fantasies about health, disease and the body" (11). In a fascinating point relevant to this study, Gilman argues that the invisible (social) fantasy of a particular illness, say insanity, was visualized through medical illustrations (18). What practitioners wanted to see in the mentally ill was ultimately depicted in seemingly representational visuals. Doctors created their own pictorial-medical proof. Freud's emphasis on the talking cure in the late-nineteenth century, Gilman thus argues, is a turn from Charcot's visual diagnosis (22). Because the field of psychiatry boosted its "visual epistemology" in concert with optical instruments like the microscope and X-ray (20), it created a taxonomy of the look of the insane, even if that look was a cultural construction repeatedly re-imagined in art (21). Kemp and Wallace show how evidence was used to support how a person's physiognomy could be scrutinized, subsequently identified and judged as primitive, criminal, amoral, uncivilized, homosexual, or insane.

8. See Anne-Emanuelle Birn's "Six Seconds per Eyelid."

9. Interestingly, Dolmage describes relevant photographs in *Disabled upon Arrival* but deposits them not inside the book but in a digital "shadow archive" at the Ohio State University Press website, "because experiencing these photographs may be difficult for some readers" (*Disabled upon Arrival* 6). He also arranges the book in a series of "snapshots, postcards, or slides" which need not be read in chronological order, as Dolmage intends "to model a disability studies methodology, an approach to history that resists normativity" ("Introduction" 5). Dolmage's innovations in, or even disruptions to, scholarship as we expect it to play out remind us that visual images recording race and/as disability are wounding; and that normative reading reproduces the status quo. Why not continue to disturb the scholarly universe, I ask.

10. Ellis Island doctors examined newcomers for signs of illness while other authorities surveilled arrivals for limps as they climbed a series of requisite stairs to the examination room, scrutinized them for odd behavior (psychological ailments), among other techniques aimed at spotting the infirm, reports Dolmage (*Disabled upon Arrival* 14).

11. See also Douglas Baynton's *Defectives in the Land* and "Disability and the Justification of Inequality in American History."

12. In a widely Western designation of Asian as alien, Mel Chen examines British physician John Langdon Down's 1866 nomenclature of Trisomy 21 as mongoloidism. Chen calls this "racial description of disability" a "colonial trope of incapacity" ("Unpacking Intoxication" 27). Also see Mark Jackson's "Changing Depictions of Disease."

13. Racism demarcated beauty as well. Unattractive snub noses among European immigrants to the US, notes Gilman, marked a subject as an Irish degenerate; a hooked nose designated a Jewish primitive (Gilman, *Picturing Health and Illness* 83, 84).

14. Moreover, if the stress of being black in America—walking down the street while black, driving while black, voting while black, shopping while black—results in increased anxiety, depression, hypertension, high blood pressure, obesity, diabetes, and heart attacks, then its

absence from the pages of graphic pathography invokes a host of inquiries that are entangled in race, representation, illness, and perhaps even shame.

15. Additionally, both *Blankets* and *Stitches* enjoy wide acclaim and a healthy existence in college classrooms; if the cartoon avatars are lost, their authors clearly are found.

16. For D. A. Miller, the practice of reading itself is ideologically constabulary: it captivates us, arrests our time, detains us in self-disciplinary reading positions. Our body also accommodates a book, so much so that certain reading postures, over time, create aches and pains. The whiteness of the pages of an empty book, then, is an ideological signifier.

Bibliography

Abate, Michelle Ann. "Art Spiegelman's *In the Shadow of No Towers* as Board Book: From the Matter of Materiality to the Way That Materiality Matters." *Jeunesse: Young People, Texts, Cultures*, vol. 7, no. 2, 2015, pp. 40–64, https://doi.org/10.1353/jeu.2015.0021. Accessed 14 June 2021.

Ahmed, Sara. *The Cultural Politics of Emotion*. Routledge, 2015.

———. *Queer Phenomenology: Orientations, Objects, Others*. Duke UP, 2006.

Akomolafe, Bayo. "I, Coronavirus. Mother. Monster. Activist." May 15, 2020, https://bayoakomolafe.net/post/i-coronavirus-mother-monster-activist/. Accessed 12 June 2020.

Alaniz, José. *Death, Disability, and the Superhero: The Silver Age and Beyond*. UP of Mississippi, 2014.

Alexander, Jeffrey C., et al., editors. *Cultural Trauma and Collective Identity*. U of California P, 2004.

Avrahami, Einat. *The Invading Body: Reading Illness Autobiographies*. U of Virginia P, 2007.

Azab, Andrew. "Feedback." Penn State Collection of Graphic Narratives, 2018, https://sites.psu.edu/graphicnarratives/2018/08/13/andrew-azab/. Accessed 1 May 2022.

B., David. *Epileptic*. Pantheon, 2005.

Bachelard, Gaston. *The Poetics of Space*. 1958. Translated by Maria Jolas. Beacon Press, 1994.

Baetens, Jan, and Hugo Frey. *The Graphic Novel: An Introduction*. Cambridge UP, 2014.

Ball, Rachael. *The Inflatable Woman*. Bloomsbury Publishing, 2015.

Banbury, Trey. "Perspective," Penn State Collection of Graphic Narratives, 2013, https://sites.psu.edu/graphicnarratives/2016/08/01/trey-banbury/. Accessed 2 Mar. 2022.

Banner, Oliva. "Structural Racism and Practices of Reading in the Medical Humanities." *Literature and Medicine*, vol. 34, no. 1, spring 2016, pp. 25–52, https://muse-jhu-edu.unh.idm.oclc.org/pub/1/article/629001/pdf. Accessed 25 Feb. 2022.

Barnes, Elizabeth. *The Minority Body: A Theory of Disability*. Oxford UP, 2016.

Baruch, Jay. "In Defense of Cheaper Stethoscopes." *Health Humanities Reader*, edited by Therese Jones, Delese Wear, and Lester D. Friedman, Rutgers UP, 2014, pp. 511–15.

Baynton, Douglas C. *Defectives in the Land: Disability and Immigration in the Age of Eugenics*. U of Chicago P, 2016.

———. "Disability and the Justification of Inequality in American History." *The Disability Studies Reader*, edited by Lennard J. Davis, 5th ed., Routledge, 2016, pp. 17–34. Google Books. Accessed 6 Feb. 2022.

Beaty, Bart. *Comics Versus Art*. U of Toronto P, 2012.

Beaty, Bart, and Benjamin Woo. *The Greatest Comic Book of All Time: Symbolic Capital and the Field of American Comic Books*. Palgrave Pivot, 2016.

Bell, Chris. "Introducing White Disability Studies: A Modest Proposal." *The Disability Studies Reader*, edited by Lennard J. Davis, 2nd ed., Routledge, 2006, pp. 275–81.

Bell, Christopher M. "Introduction: Doing Representational Detective Work." *Blackness and Disability: Critical Examinations and Cultural Interventions*, edited by Christopher Bell, Michigan State UP, 2011, pp. 1–7.
Bennett, Jane. *Influx and Efflux: Writing Up with Walt Whitman*. Duke UP, 2020.
———. *Vibrant Matter: A Political Ecology of Things*. Duke UP, 2010.
Bennett, Juda, and Cassandra Jackson. "Graphic Whiteness and the Lessons of Chris Ware's *Jimmy Corrigan*." *ImageText: Interdisciplinary Comics Studies*, vol. 5, no. 1, 2009, http://imagetext.english.ufl.edu/archives/v5_1/bennett-jackson/. Accessed 25 June 2020.
Bennett, Marek. *The Civil War Diary of Freeman Colby, 1863*, vol. 2, Comics Workshop, 2019.
Berlant, Lauren. "Cruel Optimism." *The Affect Theory Reader*, edited by Melissa Gregg and Gregory J. Seigworth, Duke UP, 2010, pp. 93–117.
Bernstein, Barbara. "Drawing a Breath." *Drawing in the Twenty-First Century: The Politics and Poetics of Contemporary Practice*, edited by Elizabeth A. Pergam, Ashgate, 2015, pp. 90–99.
Best, Stephen, and Sharon Marcus. "Surface Reading: An Introduction." *Representations*, vol. 108, no. 1, fall 2009, pp. 1–20.
Birn, Anne-Emanuelle. "Six Seconds per Eyelid: The Medical Inspection of Immigrants at Ellis Island, 1892–1914." *Dynamis*, vol. 17, 1997, pp. 281–316.
Bleakley, Alan. *Medical Humanities and Medical Education: How the Medical Humanities Can Shape Better Doctors*. Routledge, 2015.
Boileau, Kendra, and Rich Johnson, editors. *COVID Chronicles: A Comics Anthology*. Graphic Mundi, 2021.
Bolaki, Stella. "Challenging Invisibility, Making Connections: Illness, Survival, and Black Struggles in Audre Lorde's Work." *Blackness and Disability: Critical Examinations and Cultural Interventions*, edited by Christopher M. Bell, LIT Verlag, 2011, pp. 47–74.
Bordo, Susan. *Unbearable: Feminism, Western Culture, and the Body*. 2nd ed., U of California P, 2004.
Bourdieu, Pierre, and Löic J. D. Wacquant. *An Invitation to Reflexive Sociology*. U of Chicago P, 1992.
Bramlett, Frank, editor. *Linguistics and the Study of Comics*. Palgrave Macmillan, 2012.
Bredehoft, Thomas A. "Style, Voice, and Authorship in Harvey Pekar's (Auto) (Bio)Graphical Comics." *College Literature*, vol. 38, no. 3, summer 2011, pp. 97–110.
Brophy, Sarah, and Janice Hladki. "Connective Tissue: Summoning the Spectator to Visual Autobiography." *Embodied Politics in Visual Autobiography*, edited by Brophy and Hladki, U of Toronto P, 2014, pp. 244–67.
Bukatman, Scott. *Hellboy's World: Comics and Monsters on the Margins*. U of California P, 2016.
Burkart, Roland. *Twister*. Graphic Mundi, 2021.
Burke, Thomas Patrick. *The Concept of Justice? Is Justice Just?* Continuum, 2011.
Burns, Charles. *Black Hole*. Pantheon, 2008.
Butler, Judith. *Bodies That Matter: On the Discursive Limits of Sex*. Routledge, 2011.
———. *Gender Trouble: Feminism and the Subversion of Identity*. Routledge, 1990.
Capeheart, Loretta, and Dragan Milovanovic. *Social Justice: Theories, Issues, and Movements*. Revised and expanded edition. Rutgers UP, 2020.
Cartwright, Lisa. *Screening the Body: Tracing Medicine's Visual Culture*. U of Minnesota P, 1995.
Chaney, Michael A. *Reading Lessons in Seeing: Mirrors, Masks, and Mazes in the Autobiographical Graphic Novel*. UP of Mississippi, 2017.
Charon, Rita. "Introduction." *The Principles and Practice of Narrative Medicine*, edited by Rita Charon et al., Oxford UP, 2017, pp. 1–12.
———. *Narrative Medicine: Honoring the Stories of Illness*. Oxford UP, 2006.
Chast, Roz. *Can't We Talk About Something More Pleasant?* Bloomsbury USA, 2014.
———. *Going into Town: A Love Letter to New York*. Bloomsbury USA, 2017.
Chen, Mel Y. "*Animacies: Biopolitics, Racial Mattering, and Queer Affect*. Duke UP, 2012.
———. Unpacking Intoxication, Racialising Disability." *Medical Humanities*, vol. 41, no. 1, 2015, n.p., http://mh.bmj.com/. Accessed 13 Feb. 2022.

Chevely, Lyn, and Joyce Farmer. *Tits and Clits Comix*. Nanny Goat and Last Gasp, 1972–87.
Chiu, Monica, and Jeanette Roan. "Asian American Graphic Narrative." *The Oxford Encyclopedia of Asian American and Pacific Islander Literature and Culture*, edited by Josephine Lee and Floyd Cheung, Oxford UP, 2018, https://doi.org/10.1093/acrefore/9780190201098.013.784. Accessed 20 Nov. 2021.
Chong, Vivian (author and artist), and Georgia Webber (artist). *Dancing After TEN*. Fantagraphics, 2020.
Chute, Hillary L. "Comics as Literature? Reading Graphic Narrative." *PMLA*, vol. 123, no. 2, Mar. 2008, pp. 452–65.
———. "Comics Form and Narrating Lives." *Profession*, 2011, pp. 107–17, https://www.jstor.org/stable/41714112. Accessed 14 June 2021.
———. *Disaster Drawn: Visual Witness, Comics, and Documentary Form*. Harvard UP, 2016.
———. *Graphic Women: Life Narrative and Contemporary Comics*. Columbia UP, 2010.
———. Review of *Cancer Vixen. Literature and Medicine*, vol. 26, no. 5, fall 2007, pp. 413–29.
Clare, Eli. *Brilliant Imperfection: Grappling with Cure*. Duke UP, 2017.
Cohn, Neil. *The Visual Language of Comics: Introduction to the Structure and Cognition of Sequential Images*. Bloomsbury Academic, 2014.
Cole, Thomas R., Nathan S. Carlin, and Ronald A. Carson. *Medical Humanities: An Introduction*, vol. 1, Cambridge UP, 2015.
Coope, Jonathan. "On the Needs for an Ecologically Dimensioned Medical Humanities." *Journal of Medical Humanities*, vol. 47, no. 1, Mar. 2021, pp. 123–27, https://mh.bmj.com/content/medhum/47/1/123.full.pdf. Accessed 17 Dec. 2021.
Cooper, Melinda E. *Life as Surplus: Biotechnology and Capitalism in the Neoliberal Era*. U of Washington P, 2008.
Couser, G. Thomas. "Is There a Body in This Text? Embodiment in Graphic Somatography." *a/b: Autobiography Studies*, vol. 33, no. 2, 2018, pp. 347–73.
———. *Memoir: An Introduction*. Oxford UP, 2011.
———. *Recovering Bodies: Illness, Disability, and Life Writing*. U of Wisconsin P, 1997.
———. *Signifying Bodies: Disability in Contemporary Life Writing*. U of Michigan P, 2009.
———. *Vulnerable Subjects: Ethics and Life Writing*. Cornell UP, 2003.
Crang, Michael, and Nigel Thrift. "Introduction." *Thinking Space*, edited by Crang and Thrift, Routledge, 2000, pp. 2–30.
Crawford, Paul, Brian Brown et al., editors. *Health Humanities*. Palgrave Macmillan, 2015.
Cressman, Jodi. "The Embodied Witness of Graphic Pathology." *Graphic Embodiments: Perspectives on Health and Embodiment in Graphic Narratives*, edited by Jodi Cressman and Lisa DeTora, Leuven UP, 2021, pp. 23–30, https://www.jstor.org/stable/j.ctv1ccbg8p.5. Accessed 11 July 2021.
Crilley, Mariah. "Drawing Disability: Superman, Huntington's, and the Comic Form in *It's a Bird. . . .*" *Disability in Comic Books and Graphic Narratives*, edited by Chris Foss, Jonathan W. Gray, and Zach Whalen, Palgrave Macmillan, 2016, pp. 80–94.
Critical Inquiry, vol. 28, no. 1, 2001.
Czerwiec, MK, "The Crayon Revolution." *Graphic Medicine Manifesto*, edited by MK Czerwiec, Ian Williams, Susan Merrill Squier et al., Pennsylvania State UP, 2015, pp. 143–63.
———, editor. *Menopause: A Comic Treatment*. Pennsylvania State UP, 2020.
———. *Taking Turns: Stories from HIV/AIDS Care Unit 371*. Pennsylvania State UP, 2017.
Czerwiec, MK, and Michelle N. Huang. "Hospice Comics: Representations of Patient and Family Experience of Illness and Death in Graphic Novels." *Journal of Medical Humanities*, vol. 38, 2017, pp. 95–113.
Czerwiec, MK, Ian Williams, Susan Merrill Squier et al. *Graphic Medicine Manifesto*. Pennsylvania State UP, 2015.
Dahl, Ken. *Monsters*. Secret Acres, 2008.
Davis-McElligatt, Joanna. "Confronting the Intersections of Race, Immigration, and Representation in Chris Ware's Comics." *The Comics of Chris Ware*, edited by David M. Ball and Martha B. Kuhlman, UP of Mississippi, 2010, pp. 135–45.
Davison, Al. *Hokusai: Demons—and Other Tales of the Fox Mother*. Astral Gypsy, 2009.

———. Interview with Alex Fitch. "Panel Borders: *Doctor Who* and *The Spiral Cage*." Podcast. British Mavericks, 13 Nov. 2009, https://panelborders.wordpress.com/2009/11/13/panel-borders-doctor-who-and-the-spiral-cage/. Accessed 22 Jan. 2018.

———. *The Minotaur's Tale*. Orion Publishing, 1992.

———. *The Spiral Cage: Diary of an Astral Gypsy*. Expanded version. Titan, 1994.

———. *The Spiral Cage: Diary of an Astral Gypsy*. Renegade, 1988.

———. *The Spiral Cage*. Reissue. Active Images, 2003.

DeFalco, Amelia. "Graphic Somatography: Life Writing, Comics, and the Ethics of Care." *Journal of Medical Humanities*, vol. 37, 2016, pp. 223–40, https://link.Springer.com/article/10.1007/s10912-015-9360-6. Accessed 24 Sept. 2021.

del Pont, Xavier Marcó. "Confronting the Whiteness: Blankness, Loss and Visual Disintegration in Graphic Narratives." *Studies in Comics*, vol. 3, no. 2, Dec. 2021, pp. 253–74, https://doi.org/10.1386/stic.3.2.253_1. Accessed 8 June 2021.

De Souza, Luisa. "The Honors Game." 2020, https://sites.psu.edu/graphicnarratives/files/2020/04/Luisa-De-Souza-v2-on-web.pdf. Accessed 2 Mar. 2022.

DeTora, Lisa, and Jodi Cressman. "Introduction." *Graphic Embodiments: Perspectives on Health and Embodiment in Graphic Narratives*, edited by Jodi Cressman and Lisa DeTora, Leuven UP, 2021, pp. 13–20, https://doi.org/10.2307/j.ctv1ccbg8p.4. Accessed 11 July 2021.

Devlieger, Patrick, Beatriz Miranda-Galarza et al., "Introducing disABILITY MUNDUS: History, Critical Theory, and Plurality Through the Lens of Disability Culture." *Rethinking Disability: World Perspectives in Culture and Society*, edited by Patrick Devlieger, Beatriz Miranda-Galarza et al., Garant, 2016, pp. 13–22.

Diamond, Aidan, and Lauranne Poharec. "Introduction: Freaked and Other Bodies in Comics." *Journal of Graphic Novels and Comics*, vol. 8, no. 5, 2017, pp. 402–17.

Dillon, Glyn. *The Nao of Brown*. Abrams, 2012.

Dolmage, Jay. *Disabled upon Arrival: Eugenics, Immigration, and the Construction of Race and Disability*. Ohio State UP, 2018, https://www.jstor.org/stable/j.ctv1h45mm5. Accessed 14 Feb. 2022.

———. "Disabled upon Arrival: The Rhetorical Construction of Disability and Race at Ellis Island." *Cultural Critique*, vol. 77, winter 2011, pp. 24–69, https://www.jstor.org/stable/10.5749/culturalcritique.77.2011.002. Accessed 14 Feb. 2022.

Dolmage, Jay, and Dale Jacobs. "Mutable Articulations: Disability Rhetoric and the Comics Medium." *Disability in Comic Books and Graphic Narratives*, edited by Chris Foss, Jonathan W. Gray, and Zach Whalen, Palgrave Macmillan, 2016, pp. 14–28.

Dong, Lan. "The Model Minority Between Medical School and Nintendo: Gene Luen Yang and Thien Pham's *Level Up*." *Drawing New Color Lines: Transnational Asian American Graphic Narratives*, edited by Monica Chiu, Hong Kong UP, 2015, pp. 69–86.

Donovan, Courtney. "Graphic Pathogeographies." *Journal of Medical Humanities*, vol. 35, no. 3, Sept. 2014, pp. 273–99, https://doi.org/10.1007/s10912-014-9295-3. Accessed 8 June 2021.

Donovan, Courtney, and Ebru Ustundag. "Graphic Narratives, Trauma and Social Justice." *Studies in Social Justice*, vol. 11, no. 2, 2017, pp. 221–37.

Doucet, Julie. *My New York Diary*. Drawn and Quarterly, 2010.

Durand, Élodie. *Parenthesis*. Top Shelf Productions, 2021.

Edelman, Lee. *No Future: Queer Theory and the Death Drive*. Duke UP, 2004.

Eisner, Will. *Comics and Sequential Art: Principles and Practices from the Legendary Cartoonist*. W. W. Norton, 2008.

El Refaie, Elisabeth. *Visual Metaphor and Embodiment in Graphic Illness Narratives*. Oxford UP, 2019. Oxford Scholarship Online, https://doi.org/10.1093/oso/9780190678173.001.0001. Accessed 15 Jan. 2022.

Engelberg, Miriam. *Cancer Made Me a Shallower Person*. HarperCollins, 2006.

Espé (Sebastien Portret). *The Parakeet*. Translated by Hannah Chute. Graphic Mundi, 2021.

Fairfield, Lesley. *Tyranny*. Tundra Books, 2009.

Farmer, Joyce. *Special Exits: A Graphic Memoir*. Fantagraphics, 2010.

Farmer, Joyce (Joyce Sutton), and Lyn Chevely. *Abortion Eve*. Roe v. Wade Decision Comic Books, 1973, http://www.ep.tc/eve/index.html. Accessed 1 June 2021.

Farmer, Joyce, Lyn Chevely et al., editors. *Wimmen's Comix*. Last Gasp, 1972–85.

Fawaz, Ramzi. *The New Mutants: Superheroes and the Radical Imagination of American Comics*. New York UP, 2016.

Ferraro, Antonio J. "The Many Fictions of Illness: A Rhetorical Approach to Understanding Fictionality in *Mom's Cancer*." *Literature and Medicine*, vol. 39, no. 2, fall 2021, pp. 227–48.

———. "The Price of an Ending: Reading Graphic Embodiment in *Cancer Vixen*." *Graphic Embodiments: Perspectives on Health and Embodiment in Graphic Narratives*, edited by Jodi Cressman and Lisa DeTora, Leuven UP, 2021, pp. 153–62, https://www.jstor.org/stable/j.ctv1ccbg8p.15. Accessed 11 July 2021.

Fies, Brian. *Mom's Cancer*. Abrams ComicArts, 2006.

Flowers, Ebony. *Hot Comb*. Drawn & Quarterly, 2019.

Fong, Harmon. http://www.medthics.com/comics/07/07.html#page/2. Accessed 18 Mar. 2022.

Foss, Chris. "Reading in Pictures: Re-visioning Autism and Literature in the Medium of Manga." *Disability in Comic Books and Graphic Narratives*, edited by Chris Foss, Jonathan W. Gray, and Zach Whalen, Palgrave Macmillan, 2016, pp. 95–110.

Frank, Arthur W. *The Wounded Storyteller: Body, Illness, and Ethics*. U of Chicago P, 1995.

Gardner, Jared. "Beyond Metaphor." Keynote. Comics and Medicine Conference. Riverside, California, Oct. 2015, https://www.graphicmedicine.org/jared-gardner-beyond-metaphor/. Accessed 9 Nov. 2019.

———. "Storylines." *SubStance*, vol. 40, no. 1, issue 124, 2011, pp. 53–69, https://www.jstor.org/stable/41300188. Accessed 25 Sept. 2021.

Garland-Thomson, Rosemarie. "Foreword." *Disability in Comic Books and Graphic Narratives*, edited by Chris Foss, Jonathan W. Gray, and Zach Whalen. Palgrave Macmillan, UK, 2003, pp. x–xiii.

———. "The Politics of Staring: Visual Rhetorics of Disability in Popular Photography." *Disability Studies: Enabling the Humanities*, edited by Sharon L. Snyder, MLA, 2002, pp. 56–75.

———. *Staring: How We Look*. Oxford UP, 2009.

Genette, Gérard. *Palimpsests: Literature in the Second Degree*. Translated by Channa Newman and Claude Doubinsky. U of Nebraska P, 1997.

Gibbs, Anna. "After Affect: Sympathy, Synchrony, and Mimetic Communication." *The Affect Theory Reader*, edited by Melissa Gregg and Gregory J. Seigworth, Duke UP, 2010, pp. 186–205.

Gilman, Sander L. *Making the Body Beautiful: A Cultural History of Aesthetic Surgery*. Princeton UP, 1999.

———. *Picturing Health and Illness: Images of Identity and Difference*. Johns Hopkins UP, 1995.

———. *Seeing the Insane: A Visual and Cultural History of Our Attitudes Toward the Mentally Ill*. Echo Point Books and Media, 2014.

Gilman, Sander L., Hugh W. Diamond, and John Conolly. *The Face of Madness: Hugh W. Diamond and the Origin of Psychiatric Photography*. Echo Point Books and Media, 2014.

Glazer, Susan. "Graphic Medicine: Comics Turn a Critical Eye on Health Care." *The Hastings Center Report*, vol. 45, no. 3, May/June 2015, pp. 15–19.

Glenn, Evelyn Nakano. *Forced to Care: Coercion and Caregiving in America*. Harvard UP, 2012.

Goethals, Tina, Elisabeth De Schauwer, and Geert Van Hove. "Weaving Intersectionality into Disability Studies Research: Inclusion, Reflexivity and Anti-Essentialism." *DiGeSt: Journal of Diversity and Gender Studies*, vol. 2, nos. 1–2, 2015, pp. 75–94, https://www.jstor.org/stable/pdf/10.11116/jdivegendstud.2.1-2.0075.pdf. Accessed 1 Feb. 2022.

Goffman, Erving. *Stigma: Notes on the Management of Spoiled Identity*. Reissue. Touchstone, 1986.

Goto, Hiromi. *Chorus of Mushrooms*. NeWest, 1994.

Goto, Hiromi (author), and Ann Xu (artist). *Shadow Life*. First Second, 2021.

Gravett, Paul. Interview with Glyn Dillon. http://paulgravett.com/articles/article/glyn_dillon. Accessed 26 Jan. 2022.
Green, Justin. *Binky Brown Meets the Holy Virgin Mary*. 1972. McSweeney's Books, 2009.
Green, Katie. *Lighter Than My Shadow*. Jonathan Cape/Vintage, 2013.
Green, Michael J. "Graphic Storytelling and Medical Narrative: The Use of Comics in Medical Education." *Graphic Medicine Manifesto*, MK Czerwiec, Ian Williams, Susan Merrill Squier et al., Pennsylvania State UP, 2005, pp. 67–86.
Green, Michael J., and Kimberly R. Myers. "Graphic Medicine: Use of Comics in Medical Education and Patient Care." *BMJ*, vol. 340, no. 3 Mar. 2010, n.p., https://doi.org/10.1136/bmj.c863. Accessed 17 June 2020.
Gries, Laurie. *Still Life with Rhetoric: A New Materialist Approach for Visual Rhetorics*. Utah State UP, 2015.
Groensteen, Thierry. *Comics and Narration*. Translated by Ann Miller. UP of Mississippi, 2013.
———. *The System of Comics*. Translated by Bart Beaty and Nick Nguyen. UP of Mississippi, 2007.
Guibert, Emmanuel (artist), Didier Lefèvre (photographer), and Frédéric Lemercier (colorist). *The Photographer: Into War-Torn Afghanistan with Doctors Without Borders*. Translated by Alexis Siegel. First Second, 2009.
Gumbs, Alexis Pauline. "M/other Ourselves: A Black Queer Feminist Genealogy for Radical Mothering." *Revolutionary Mothering: Love on the Front Lines*, edited by Alexis Pauline Gumbs, China Martens, and Mai'a Williams, PM Press, 2016, pp. 19–35.
Hansen, Bert. "Medical History's Graphic Power in American True-Adventure Comic Books of the 1940s." *Handbook of Popular Culture and Biomedicine: Knowledge in the Life Sciences as Cultural Artefact*, edited by Arno Görgen, German Alfonso Nunez, Heiner Fangerau, Springer International Publishing AG, 2019, pp. 179–94.
Harvey, Robert C. *The Art of the Comic Book: An Aesthetic*. UP of Mississippi, 1996.
Hatfield, Elaine, John T. Cacioppo, and Richard L. Rapson. *Emotional Contagion*. Cambridge UP, 1993.
Hawkins, Anne Hunsaker. *Reconstructing Illness: Studies in Pathography*. Purdue UP, 1999.
Hawkins, Anne Hunsaker, and Marilyn Chandler McEntyre. "Introduction: Teaching Literature and Medicine: A Retrospective and a Rationale." *Teaching Literature and Medicine*, edited by Anne Hunsaker Hawkins and Marilyn Chandler McEntyre, MLA, 2000, pp. 1–25.
Hayden, Jennifer. *The Story of My Tits*. Top Shelf Productions, 2015.
Heinrich, Ari Larissa. *The Afterlife of Images: Translating the Pathological Body Between China and the West*. Duke UP, 2008.
Herndl, Diane Price. "Disease Versus Disability: The Medical Humanities and Disability Studies." *PMLA*, vol. 120, no. 2, Mar. 2005, pp. 593–98.
———. *Invalid Women: Figuring Feminine Illness in American Fiction and Culture, 1840–1940*. U of North Carolina P, 1993.
Holmes. "Good People Great Medicine." 2016, https://bpb-us-e1.wpmucdn.com/sites.psu.edu/dist/e/58355/files/2016/08/Holmes.pdf. Accessed 18 Apr. 2023.
Holmes, Martha Stoddard. "Cancer Comics: Narrating Cancer Through Sequential Art." *Tulsa Studies in Women's Literature*, vols. 32/33, nos. 2/3, fall 2013/spring 2014, pp. 147–62.
Hunter, Kathryn Montgomery. *Doctors' Stories: The Narrative Structure of Medical Knowledge*. Princeton UP, 1991.
Jackson, Cassandra. "Visualizing Slavery: Photography and the Disabled Subject in the Art of Carrie Mae Weems." *Blackness and Disability: Critical Examinations and Cultural Interventions*, edited by Christopher M. Bell, Michigan State UP, 2011, pp. 31–46.
Jackson, Mark. "Changing Depictions of Disease: Race, Representation and the History of Mongolism." *Race, Science, and Medicine, 1700–1960*, edited by Waltraud Ernst and Bernard Harris, Routledge, 1999, pp. 167–88.
James, Jennifer C., and Cynthia Wu. "Editor's Introduction: Race, Ethnicity, Disability, and Literature: Intersections and Interventions." *MELUS*, vol. 31, no. 3, fall 2006, pp. 3–13.
Jenkins, Henry. *Comics and Stuff*. New York UP, 2020.

Jones, Therese, Delese Wear, and Lester D. Friedman. "Introduction: The Why, the What, and the How of the Medical/Health Humanities." *Health Humanities Reader*, edited by Therese Jones, Delese Wear, and Lester D. Friedman, Rutgers UP, 2014, pp. 1–11.

Jordanova, Ludmilla. "Medicine and the Visual Arts: Overview." *Medicine, Health and the Arts*, edited by Victoria Bates, Alan Bleakley, and Sam Goodman, Routledge, 2014, pp. 41–63.

———. *Sexual Visions: Images of Gender in Science and Medicine Between the Eighteenth and Twentieth Centuries*. U of Wisconsin P, 1993.

Jurecic, Ann. *Illness as Narrative*. U of Pittsburgh P, 2012.

Kasthuri, Raghavi Ravi, and Anu Mary Peter. "Twelve Years of Graphic Medicine: A Conversation with Comic Nurse on the Future of Comics and Medicine." *Configurations*, vol. 29, no. 1, winter 2021, pp. 97–106.

Kemp, Martin, and Marina Wallace. *Spectacular Bodies: The Art and Science of the Human Body from Leonardo to Now*. U of California P, 2000.

King, Samantha. *Pink Ribbons, Inc.: Breast Cancer and the Politics of Philanthropy*. U of Minnesota P, 2006.

Kirtley, Susan E. *Lynda Barry: Girlhood Through the Looking Glass*. UP of Mississippi, 2012.

Kittay, Eva Feder. *Love's Labor: Essays on Women, Equality and Dependency*. 2nd ed., Routledge, 2019.

Kleinman, Arthur. *The Illness Narratives: Suffering, Healing, and the Human Condition*. Perseus, 1988.

Klugman, Craig, Jennifer Peel, and Diane Beckmann-Mendez. "Making the Rounds: Art Rounds: Teaching Interprofessional Students Visual Thinking Strategies at One School." *Academic Medicine*, vol. 86, no. 10, Oct. 2011, https://doi.org/10.1097/ACM.0b013e31822c1427. Accessed 22 Jan. 2022.

Knisley, Lucy. *Displacement: A Travelogue*. Fantagraphics, 2015.

Koch, Christina Maria. "Comic-Grotesque Metamorphoses: Boundaries Between Illness and Health in Ken Dahl's *Monsters*." *Comics an der Grenze: Sub/Versionen von Form und Inhalt*, edited by Matthias Harbeck, Linda-Rabea Heyden, and Marie Schröer, Verlag, 2017, pp. 149–64.

Køhlert, Frederik Byrn. "'A Grotesque, Incurable Disease': Whiteness as Illness in Gabby Schultz's *Sick*." *Inks: The Journal of the Comics Studies Society*, vol. 4, no. 2, summer 2020, pp. 199–220, https://muse-jhu-edu.unh.idm.oclc.org/pub/30/article/764587. Accessed 28 Feb. 2022.

———. *Serial Selves: Identity and Representation in Autobiographical Comics*. Rutgers UP, 2019.

Kulick, Don, and Jens Rydström. *Loneliness and Its Opposite: Sex, Disability, and the Ethics of Engagement*. Duke UP, 2016.

Kumagai, Arno K., and Monica L. Lypson. "Beyond Cultural Competence: Critical Consciousness, Social Justice, and Multicultural Education." *Academic Medicine*, vol. 84, no. 6, June 2009, pp. 782–87, https://doi.org/10.1097/ACM.0b013e3181a42398. Accessed 1 Mar. 2022.

Kunka, Andrew. *Autobiographical Comics*. Bloomsbury Academic, 2018.

Lakoff, George, and Mark Johnson. *Metaphors We Live By*. U of Chicago P, 2003.

Laqueur, Thomas. *Making Sex: Gender and the Body from the Greeks to Freud*. Harvard UP, 1992.

Launer, John. *Narrative-Based Primary Care: A Practical Guide*. 1st ed., CRC Press, 2002.

Lavin, Shane. "Whatever Floats Your Boat," https://sites.psu.edu/graphicnarratives/wp-content/uploads/sites/58355/2016/08/Shane-Lavin.pdf. 2012. Accessed 1 Mar. 2022.

Leavitt, Sarah. *Tangles: A Story About Alzheimer's, My Mother, and Me*. Skyhorse, 2012.

Leder, Drew. *The Absent Body*. U of Chicago P, 1990.

Lee, James Kyung-Jin. *Pedagogies of Woundedness: Illness, Memoir, and the Ends of the Model Minority*. Temple UP, 2022.

Lee, Rachel C. *The Exquisite Corpse of Asian America: Biopolitics, Biosociality, and Posthuman Ecologies*. New York UP, 2014.

Lefebvre, Henri. *The Production of Space*. Translated by Donald Nicholson-Smith. Wiley-Blackwell, 1992.

Lehrer, Riva. "Consent to Be Seen." Exhibition. Haverford College, 2016–17, https://courtneylynnecarter.wordpress.com/exhibitions/. Accessed 16 Jan. 2022.

Linton, Simi. *Claiming Disability: Knowledge and Identity*. New York UP, 1998, https://ebookcentral.proquest.com/lib/unh/reader.action?docID=865773. Accessed 22 April 2023.

Lorde, Audre. *The Cancer Journals*. Spinsters Ink, 1980.

Lorenz, Walter. Untitled. *Routledge International Handbook of Social Justice*, edited by Michael Reisch, Routledge, 2016, pp. 13–26.

Love, Heather. *Feeling Backward: Loss and the Politics of Queer History*. Harvard UP, 2009.

Lye, Colleen. *America's Asia: Racial Form and American Literature, 1893–1945*. Princeton UP, 2004.

Mack, Stan. *Janet and Me: An Illustrated Story of Love and Loss*. Simon & Shuster, 2004.

Magnet, Shoshona, and Amanda Watson. "How to Get Through the Day with Pain and Sadness: Temporality and Disability in Graphic Novels." *Disability Media Studies*, edited by Elizabeth Ellcessor and Bill Kirkpatrick, New York UP, 2017, pp. 247–74.

Magnus, Kathy Dow. "The Unaccountable Subject: Judith Butler and the Social Conditions of Intersubjective Agency." *Hypatia*, vol. 21, no. 2, spring 2006, pp. 81–103, https://www.jstor.org/stable/3810993. Accessed 25 Jan. 2022.

Marchetto, Marisa Acocella. *Ann Tenna*. 1st ed., Alfred A. Knopf, 2015.

———. *Cancer Vixen: A True Story*. Reprint. Pantheon, 2009.

Martin, Emily. *The Woman in the Body: A Cultural Analysis of Reproduction*. Beacon Press, 2001.

McCloud, Scott. *Understanding Comics: The Invisible Art*. HarperCollins, 1994.

McGuire, Richard. *Here*. Pantheon, 2014.

McIlvenny, Paul. "Disabling Men: Masculinity and Disability in Al Davison's Graphic Autobiography *The Spiral Cage*." *Bending Bodies: Moulding Masculinities*, edited by Søren Edvø and Thomas Johansson, vol. 2, Ashgate, 2003, pp. 238–58.

Menakem, Resmaa. *My Grandmother's Hands: Racialized Trauma and the Pathways to Mending Our Hearts and Bodies*. Central Recovery P, 2017.

Metz, Jonathan M., and Anna Kirkland, editors. *Against Health: How Health Became the New Morality*. New York UP, 2010.

Mikkonen, Kai. "Subjectivity and Style in Graphic Narratives." *From Comic Strips to Graphic Novels: Contributions to the Theory and History of the Graphic Narrative*, edited by Daniel Stein and Jan-Noël Thon, De Gruyter, 2105, pp. 101–23. Proquest Ebook Central, https://ebookcentral.proquest.com/lib/unh/reader.action?docID=2035737&ppg=31. Accessed 24 Jan. 2021.

Miller, D. A. *The Novel and the Police*. U of California P, 1989.

Miller, Daniel. *Stuff*. 1st ed., Polity, 2009.

Miller, Frank. *Batman: The Dark Night Returns*. DC Comics, 1986.

Mingus, Mia. "Access Intimacy: The Missing Link." 5 May 2011, https://leavingevidence.wordpress.com/2011/05/05/access-intimacy-the-missing-link/. Accessed 25 Feb. 2022.

Miodrag, Hannah. *Comics and Language: Reimagining Critical Discourse on the Form*. UP of Mississippi, 2013.

Mirzoeff, Nicholas. *The Right to Look: A Counterhistory of Visuality*. Duke UP, 2011.

Mitchell, David T., and Sharon L. Snyder. "Preface: Mapping Identity: Disability and Other 'Marked' Bodies." *Narrative Prosthesis: Disability and the Dependencies of Discourse*, edited by David T. Mitchell and Sharon L. Snyder, U of Michigan P, 2001, pp. ix–xviii.

Molotiu, Andrei. "List of Terms for Comics Studies." *Comics Forum*, https://comicsforum.org/2013/07/26/list-of-terms-for-comics-studies-by-andrei-molotiu/. Accessed 2 July 2021.

Monk, Jeffrey. "A Ghost of an Idea," 2016, https://sites.psu.edu/graphicnarratives/2016/08/01/jefferey-monk/. Accessed 16 Mar. 2022.

Montgomery, Kathryn. *How Doctors Think: Clinical Judgment and the Practice of Medicine*. Oxford UP, 2006.

Moore, Alan (author), Dave Gibbons (artist/letterer), and John Higgins (colorist). *Watchmen*. 1986, 1987. DC Comics, 2020.

Mullins, Katie. "Embodiment, Time, and the Life Review in Jeff Lemire's *Ghost Stories*. *ESC: English Studies in Canada*, vol. 40, no. 4, Dec. 2014, pp. 29–54, https://www.doi.org/10.1353/esc.2014.0039. Accessed 7 Feb. 2019.

Murali, Chinmay, and Sathyaraj Venkatesan. *Infertility Comics and Graphic Medicine*. Routledge, 2022.

Myers, Kimberly R. "Graphic Pathography in the Classroom and the Clinic: A Case Study." *Graphic Medicine Manifesto*, MK Czerwiec, Ian Williams, Susan Merrill Squier et al., Pennsylvania State UP, 2015, pp. 87–114.

Ngai, Sianne. *Ugly Feelings*. Harvard UP, 2005.

Nussbaum, Martha. *Poetic Justice: The Literary Imagination and Public Life*. Beacon, 1995.

O'Brien, Sharon. "Showing the Voice of the Body: Brian Fies' *Mom's Cancer*, the Graphic Illness Memoir, and the Narrative of Hope." *Drawing from Life: Memory and Subjectivity in Comic Art*, edited by Jane Tolmie, UP of Mississippi, 2013: pp. 264–87.

Obuobi, Shirlene. "Shirlywhirl, MD," https://shirlywhirlmd.com/. Accessed 2 Mar. 2022.

Orbán, Katalin. "A Language of Scratches and Stitches: The Graphic Novel Between Hyperreading and Print." *Critical Inquiry*, vol. 40, no. 3, spring 2014, pp. 169–81.

Ostherr, Kirsten. *Medical Visions: Producing the Patient Through Film, Television, and Imaging Technologies*. Oxford UP, 2013.

Ousager, Jakob, and Helle Johannessen. "Humanities in Undergraduate Medical Education: A Literature Review." *Academic Medicine: Journal of the Association of American Medical Colleges*, vol. 85, no. 6, June 2010, pp. 988–98, https://doi.org/10.1097/ACM.0b013e3181dd226b. Accessed 26 Feb. 2022.

Painter, Joe. "Pierre Bourdieu." *Thinking* Space, edited by Mike Crang and Nigel Thrift, Routledge, 2000, pp. 239–59.

Panagia, Davide. *The Political Life of Sensation*. Duke UP, 2009.

Pedri, Nancy. "Cartooning Ex-Posing Photography in Graphic Memoir." *Literature and Aesthetics*, vol. 22, no. 2, Dec. 2012, pp. 248–66, https://openjournals.library.sydney.edu.au/LA/article/view/7619. Accessed 13 Apr. 2023.

———. "Photography and the Layering of Perspective in Graphic Memoir." *ImageText: Interdisciplinary Comics Studies*, vol. 9, no. 2, 2017, n.p., http://imagetext.english.ufl.edu/archives/v9_2/pedri/. Accessed 5 June 2021.

Pedri, Nancy, and Irene Velentzas. "Sexuality and Mental Illness in Comics: Notes Toward an Introduction." *Journal of Graphic Novels and Comics*, vol. 11, no. 4, 2020, pp. 357–72.

Pekar, Harvey. *The New American Splendor Anthology: From Off the Streets of Cleveland*. Running Press Adult, 1993.

Pekar, Harvey (author), Joyce Brabner (author), and Frank Stack (artist). *Our Cancer Year*. Four Walls Eight Windows, 1994.

Polak, Kate. *Ethics in the Gutter: Empathy and Historical Fiction in Comics*. Ohio State UP, 2017.

Poo, Ai-jen. *The Age of Dignity: Preparing for the Elder Boom in a Changing America*. The New Press, 2016.

Porcellino, John. *The Hospital Suite*. Drawn & Quarterly, 2014.

Potts, Phoebe. *Good Eggs: A Memoir*. Harper, 2010.

Powell, Nate. "Nate Powell." http://www.seemybrotherdance.org/bio/. Accessed 15 June 2021.

———. *Swallow Me Whole*. Top Shelf Productions, 2008.

Puar, Jasbir K. *The Right to Maim: Debility, Capacity, Disability*. Duke UP, 2017.

Quesenberry, Krista. "Intersectional and Non-human Self-Representation in Women's Autobiographical Comics." *Journal of Graphic Novels and Comics*, vol. 8, no. 5, Sept. 2017, pp. 417–32, https://doi.org/10.1080/21504857.2017.1355831. Accessed 12 June 2020.

Riddle, Christopher A. "The Ontology of Impairment: Rethinking How We Define Disability." *Emerging Perspectives on Disability Studies*, edited by Matthew Wappett and Katrina Arndt, Palgrave Macmillan, 2013, pp. 23–39.

Roberts, Chadwick. *Tits and Clits*: Sexuality and Activism in Woman-Authored Underground Comics." *Intensities: The Journal of Cult Media*, no. 9, May 2017, pp. 18–33. https://www.intensitiescultmedia.com. Accessed 13 Apr. 2023.

Roca, Paco. *Wrinkles*. Fanfare, 2015.

Rodriguez, Ralph E. "In Plain Sight: Reading the Racial Surfaces of Adrian Tomine's *Shortcomings. Drawing New Color Lines: Transnational Asian American Graphic Narratives*, edited by Monica Chiu, Hong Kong UP, 2015, pp. 87–106.

Roher, Rebecca. *Bird in a Cage*. Conundrum Press, 2016.

Ronan, Lara K., and MK Czerwiec. "A Novel Graphic Medicine Curriculum for Resident Physicians: Boosting Empathy and Communication Through Comics." *Journal of Medical Humanities*, vol. 41, no. 4, Dec. 2020, pp. 573–78, https://link.springer.com/article/10.1007/s10912-020-09654-2. Accessed 1 Mar. 2022.

Rosand, David. *Drawing Acts: Studies in Graphic Expression and Representation*. Cambridge UP, 2002.

Sabin, Roger. *Comics, Comix and Graphic Novels: A History of Comic Art*. Phaidon, 1996.

Samuels, Ellen. *Fantasies of Identification: Disability, Gender, Race*. New York UP, 2014.

Schiebinger, Londa. *Nature's Sex: Gender in the Making of Modern Science*. Rutgers UP, 2004.

Schleifer, Ronald, Jerry Vannatta, and Sheila Crow. *The Chief Concern of Medicine: The Integration of the Medical Humanities and Narrative Knowledge into Medical Practices*. U of Michigan P, 2013, pp. 137–67. *ProQuest Ebook Central*, http://ebookcentral.proquest.com/lib/unh/detail.action?docID=3415120. Accessed 3 Oct. 2019.

Schulz, Gabby. *Sick*. 2019. Secret Acres, 2016.

Sedgwick, Eve Kosofsky. *Touching Feeling: Affect, Pedagogy, Performativity*. Duke UP, 2003.

Segal, Judy Z. "Breast Cancer Narratives as Public Rhetoric: Genre Itself and the Maintenance of Ignorance." *Linguistics and the Human Sciences*, vol. 3, no. 1, 2007, pp. 3–23, https://doi.org/10.1558/lhs.v3i1.3. Accessed 4 July 2019.

Shah, Nayan. *Contagious Divides: Epidemics and Race in San Francisco's Chinatown*. U of California P, 2001.

Sharpe, Christina. *In the Wake: On Blackness and Being*. Duke UP, 2016.

Shildrick, Margrit. *Embodying the Monster: Encounters with the Vulnerable Self*. SAGE, 2002.

Siebers, Tobin Anthony. *Disability Theory*. U of Michigan P, 2008.

Skloot, Rebecca. *The Immortal Life of Henrietta Lacks*. Crown, 2011.

Small, David. *Stitches: A Memoir*. W. W. Norton, 2009.

Soja, Edward W. *Thirdspace: Journeys to Los Angeles and Other Real-and-Imagined Places*. Blackwell Publishers, 1996.

Sontag, Susan. *Illness as Metaphor and AIDS and its Metaphors*. Reprint. Anchor, 1990.

Spandler, Helen. "Crafting Psychiatric Contention Through Single-Panel Cartoons. *PathoGraphics: Narrative, Aesthetics, Contention, Community*, edited by Susan Merrill Squier and Irmela Marei Krüger-Fürhoff, Pennsylvania State UP, 2020, pp. 115–34.

Spiegelman, Art. *Maus I: A Survivor's Tale: My Father Bleeds History*. Pantheon, 1986.

———. *Maus II: A Survivor's Tale: And Here My Troubles Began*. Reprint. Pantheon, 1992.

Spillers, Hortense J. "Mama's Baby. Papa's Maybe: An American Grammar Book." *Diacritics*, vol. 17, no. 2, summer 1987, pp. 64–81, https://www.jstor.org/stable/464747. Accessed 17 Aug. 2021.

Squier, Susan M. "Comics in the Health Humanities: A New Approach to Sex and Gender Education." *Health Humanities Reader*, edited by Therese Jones, Delese Wear, and Lester D. Friedman, Rutgers UP, 2014, pp. 226–41.

———. "Literature and Medicine, Future Tense: Making It Graphic." *Literature and Medicine*, vol. 27, no. 2, 2008, pp. 124–52.

Squier, Susan Merrill. "Scaling Graphic Medicine: The Porous Pathography, a New Kind of Illness Narrative." *PathoGraphics: Narrative, Aesthetics, Contention, Community*, edited by Susan Merrill Squier and Irmela Marei Krüger-Fürhoff, Pennsylvania State UP, 2020, pp. 205–25.

———. "The Uses of Graphic Medicine for Engaged Scholarship." *Graphic Medicine Manifesto*, MK Czerwiec, Ian Williams, Squier et al., Pennsylvania State UP, 2015, pp. 41–66.

Squier, Susan Merrill, and Irmela Marei Krüger-Fürhoff, editors. *PathoGraphics: Narrative, Aesthetics, Contention, Community*. Pennsylvania State UP, 2020.

Squier, Susan, and J. Ryan Marks. "Introduction." *Configurations*, vol. 22, no. 2, spring 2014, pp. 149–52.

Squiers, Carol. *The Body at Risk: Photography of Disorder, Illness, and Healing*. U of California P, 2006.

Stacey, Jackie. *Teratologies: A Cultural Study of Cancer*. Routledge, 1997.

Stein, Daniel, and Jan-Noël Thon, editors. *From Comic Strips to Graphic Novels: Contributions to the Theory and History of the Graphic Narrative*. De Gruyter, 2105, https://ebookcentral.proquest.com/lib/unh/readerv.action?docID=2035737. Accessed 24 Jan. 2021.

Stein, Gertrude. *The Autobiography of Alice B. Toklas*. Harcourt, Brace and Company, 1933.

Stockton, Kathryn Bond. *The Queer Child, or Growing Sideways in the Twentieth Century*. Duke UP, 2009.

Strickfaden, Megan. "In Focus: Blind Photographers Challenge Visual Expectations." *Rethinking Disability: World Perspectives in Culture and Society*, edited by Patrick Delieger et al., Garant, 2013, pp. 149–64.

Sulik, Gayle A. *Pink Ribbon Blues: How Breast Cancer Culture Undermines Women's Health*. Updated version. Oxford UP, 2012.

Szép, Eszter. *Comics and the Body: Drawing, Reading, and Vulnerability*. Ohio State UP, 2020.

Taylor, Whit. *Up Down Clown*. Ninth Art Press, 2015.

Tepper, Mitchell S. "Sexuality and Disability: The Missing Discourse of Pleasure." *Sexuality and Disability*, vol. 18, 2000, pp. 283–90.

Thompson, Craig. *Blankets*. Top Shelf Productions, 2003.

Thorogood, Zoe. *The Impending Blindness of Billie Scott*. Avery Hill, 2020.

Tobe, Keiko. *With the Light: Raising an Autistic Child*, vol. 1, Yen Press, 2016.

Tobimatsu, Kimiko (author, contributor), and Keet Geniza (artist). *Kimiko Does Cancer*. Arsenal Pulp, 2020.

Tolmie, Jane, editor. *Drawing from Life: Memory and Subjectivity in Comic Art*. UP of Mississippi, 2013.

Tolstoy, Leo. *The Death of Ivan Ilyich*. Penguin Classics, 1987.

Tomine, Adrian. *Killing and Dying*. Drawn & Quarterly, 2015.

Trautmann, Joanne. *Healing Arts in Dialogue: Medicine and Literature*. Southern Illinois UP, 1982.

Tuan, Yi-Fu. *Space and Place*. U of Minnesota P, 1977.

Turkle, Sherry. *Evocative Objects: Things We Think With*. MIT Press, 2007, https://ebookcentral.proquest.com/lib/unh/reader.action?docID=3338681. Accessed 18 Feb. 2022.

Ty, Eleanor. *The Politics of the Visible in Asian North American Narratives*. U of Toronto P, 2004.

———. *Unfastened: Globality and Asian North American Narratives*. U of Minnesota P, 2010.

Vanistendael, Judith. *When David Lost His Voice*. SelfMadeHero, 2012.

Venkatesan, Sathyaraj and Chinmay Murali. "'I Don't Even Feel Human Anymore': Monstrosity and Othering in Ken Dahl's *Monsters*." *Rupkatha Journal on Interdisciplinary Studies in the Humanities*, vol. 10, no. 3, Oct. 2018, pp. 69–81.

Venkatesan, Sathyaraj, and Anu Mary Peter. "'No Time to Rest, Vent, or Mourn': Medical Intern Narratives and Graphic Medicine." *Inks: The Journal of the Comics Studies Society*, vol. 1, no. 2, summer 2017, pp. 186–204, https://www.researchgate.net/publication/332115011_No_time_to_rest_vent_or_mourn_Medical_Intern_Narratives_and_Graphic_Medicine. Accessed 6 Jan. 2022.

Verghese, Abraham. "Culture Shock—Patient as Icon, Icon as Patient." *New England Journal of Medicine*, vol. 26, no. 359, Dec. 2008, pp. 2748–51, https://www.nejm.org. Accessed 22 Jan. 2022.

Viney, William, Felicity Callard, and Angela Woods. "Critical Medical Humanities: Embracing Entanglement, Taking Risks." *Med Humanities*, vol. 41, 2015, pp. 2–7, https://mh.bmj.com/content/41/1/2. Accessed 16 May 2020.

Wailoo, Keith. *How Cancer Crossed the Color Line*. Oxford UP, 2011. *ProQuest Ebook Central*, http://ebookcentral.proquest.com/lib/unh/detail.action?docID=737546. Accessed 2 Feb. 2022.

Walrath, Dana. *Aliceheimer's: Alzheimer's Through the Looking Glass*. Pennsylvania State UP, 2016.

Walters, Shannon. "Graphic Violence in Word and Image: Reimagining Closure in *The Ride Together*." *Disability in Comic Books and Graphic Narratives*, edited by Chris Foss, Jonathan W. Gray, and Zach Whalen, Palgrave Macmillan, 2016, pp. 111–24.
Wang, Dorothy. *Thinking Its Presence: Form, Race, and Subjectivity in Contemporary Asian American Poetry*. Stanford UP, 2015.
Wanzo, Rebecca. *The Content of Our Caricature: African American Comic Art and Political Belonging*. New York UP, 2020.
Waples, Emily. "Avatars, Illness, and Authority: Embodied Experience in Breast Cancer Autopathographics." *Configurations*, vol. 22, no. 2, spring 2014, pp. 153–81.
Ware, Chris. *Building Stories*. Pantheon, 2012.
———. *Jimmy Corrigan: The Smartest Kid on Earth*. Pantheon, 2003.
Washington, Harriet A. *Medical Apartheid: The Dark History of Medical Experimentation on Black Americans from Colonial Times to the Present*. Anchor, 2008.
Waxman, Barbara Frey. *To Live in the Center of the Moment: Literary Autobiographies of Aging*. UP of Virginia, 1997.
Wear, Delese. "The Medical Humanities: Toward a Renewed Praxis." *Journal of Medical Humanities*, vol. 30, 2009, pp. 209–20, https://doi.org/10.1007/s10912-009-9091-7. Accessed 1 Mar. 2022.
Wear, Delese, Arno K. Kumagai et al., "Cultural Competency 2.0: Exploring the Concept of 'Difference' in Engagement with the Other." *Academic Medicine*, vol. 87, no. 6, June 2012, pp. 752–58, https://doi.org/10.1097/ACM.0b013e318253cef8. Accessed 1 Mar. 2022.
Webber, Georgia. *Dumb: Living Without a Voice*. Fantagraphics, 2018.
Wegner, Gesine. "Reflections on the Boom of Graphic Pathography: The Effects and Affects of Narrating Disability and Illness in Comics." *Journal of Literary and Cultural Disability Studies*, vol. 14, no. 1, 2020, pp. 57–74.
Weheliye, Alexander G. *Habeas Viscus: Racializing Assemblages, Biopolitics, and Black Feminist Theories of the Human*. Duke UP, 2014.
Wendell, Susan. "Unhealthy Disabled: Treating Chronic Illnesses as Disabilities." *Hypatia*, vol. 16, no. 4, fall 2001, pp. 17–33.
Wertz, Julie. *Tenements, Towers and Trash: An Unconventional Illustrated History of New York City*. Black Dog & Leventhal, 2017.
Whalen, Zach, Chris Foss, and Jonathan W. Gray. "Introduction: From Feats of Clay to Narrative Prose/Thesis." *Disability in Comic Books and Graphic Narratives*, edited by Chris Foss, Jonathan W. Gray, and Zach Whalen, Palgrave Macmillan, 2016, pp. 1–13.
Whitehead, Anne. "The Medical Humanities: A Literary Perspective. Overview." *Medicine, Health and the Arts: Approaches to the Medical Humanities*, edited by Victoria Bates, Alan Bleakley, and Sam Goodman, Routledge, 2014, pp. 107–27.
Whitehead, Anne, and Angela Woods. "Introduction." *The Edinburgh Companion to Critical Medical Humanities*, edited by Sara Atkinson et al., Edinburgh UP, 2016, pp. 1–32, https://www.jstor.org/stable/10.3366/j.ctt1bgzddd.5. Accessed 11 July 2021.
Whitlock, Gillian. "Autographics: The Seeing 'I' of the Comics." *Modern Fiction Studies*, vol. 52, no. 4, 2006, pp. 965–79.
Willberg, Kriota. *Draw Stronger: Self-Care for Cartoonists and Visual Artists*. Uncivilized Books, 2018.
———. *Silver Wire*. Kriota Willberg, 2018.
Williams, Ian. *The Bad Doctor: The Troubled Life and Times of Dr. Iwan James*. Pennsylvania State UP, 2015.
———. "Comics and the Iconography of Illness." *Graphic Medicine Manifesto*, MK Czerwiec, Ian Williams, Susan Merrill Squier et al., Pennsylvania State UP, 2015, pp. 115–42.
———. *The Lady Doctor*. Pennsylvania State UP, 2019.
Williams, Ian C. M. "Graphic Medicine: The Portrayal of Illness in Underground and Autobiographical Comics. Case Study." *Medicine, Health and the Arts: Approaches to the Medical Humanities*, edited by Victoria Bates, Alan Bleakley, and Sam Goodman, Routledge, 2014, pp. 64–84.

Williams, Paul. "'A Purely American Tale': The Tragedy of Racism and *Jimmy Corrigan: The Smartest Kid on Earth* as Great America Novel." *The Rise of the American Comics Artist: Creators and Contexts*, edited by Paul Williams and James Lyons, UP of Mississippi, 2010, pp. 194–209.

Wohlmann, Anita, and Madaline Harrison. "To Be Continued: Serial Narration, Chronic Disease, and Disability." *Literature and Medicine*, vol. 37, no. 1, spring 2019, pp. 67–95.

Wong, Teresa. *Dear Scarlet: The Story of My Postpartum Depression*. Arsenal Pulp Press, 2019.

Wright, Aneurin. *Things to Do in a Retirement Home Trailer Park . . . When You're 29 and Unemployed*. Pennsylvania State UP, 2015.

Yang, Gene Luen. *Dragon Hoops: From Small Steps to Great Leaps*. First Second, 2020.

Younie, Louise. "Art in Medical Education: Practice and Dialogue. A Case Study." *Medicine, Health and the Arts: Approaches to the Medical Humanities*, edited by Victoria Bates, Alan Bleakley, and Sam Goodman, Routledge, 2014, pp. 64–84.

Zaharijević, Adriana. "On Butler's Theory of Agency." *Bodies That Still Matter: Resonances of the Work of Judith Butler*, edited by Annemie Halsema, Katja Kwastek, and Roel van den Oever, Amsterdam UP, 2021, pp. 21–30, https://www-jstor-org.unh.idm.oclc.org/stable/j.ctv1m592dp.4. Accessed 25 Jan. 2022.

Ziegler, James J. "A Secret History of Miscegenation: *Jimmy Corrigan* and the Columbian Exposition of 1893." *The Blacker the Ink: Constructions of Black Identity in Comics and Sequential Art*, edited by Frances Gatewood and John Jennings, Rutgers UP, 2015, pp. 292–313.

Index

Italicized page references indicate illustrations. Endnotes are referenced with "n" followed by the endnote number.

Milton Keynes UK
Ingram Content Group UK Ltd.
UKHW012255060324
438913UK00003B/74